CLINICS IN DEVELOPMENTAL MEDICINE NO. 90

MANAGEMENT OF THE MOTOR DISORDERS OF CHILDREN WITH CEREBRAL PALSY

Edited by

David Scrutton

1984
Spastics International Medical Publications
OXFORD: Blackwell Scientific Publications Ltd.
PHILADELPHIA: J. B. Lippincott Co.

First published 1984

British Library Cataloguing in Publication Data

Scrutton, David
    Management of the motor disorders of children with cerebral palsy—(Clinics in Developmental Medicine No. 90)
    1. Cerebral palsied children.   2. Motor learning.
    I. Title   II. Series
    155.4′516   RJ496.C4

ISBN 0-632-01294-3

Printed in Great Britain at The Lavenham Press Ltd., Lavenham, Suffolk

CONTENTS

CONTRIBUTORS

BERTA BOBATH — Director of Studies, The Bobath Centre, 5 Netherhall Gardens, London NW3 5RN.

KAREL BOBATH — Honorary Consultant Physician, The Bobath Centre, 5 Netherhall Gardens, London NW3 5RN.

BRUCE GANS — Chairman, Department of Rehabilitation Medicine, New England Medical Center, Boston.

MARIA HARI — Director of the State Institute of Conductive Education of the Motor Disabled, Conductor's College, Budapest.

GEORGE JESIEN — Outreach Director, The Portage Project, Portage, Wisconsin.

LINDSAY McLELLAN — Europe Professor of Rehabilitation, Southampton University; Honorary Consultant Neurologist, Portsmouth and Southampton Health Districts.

DAVID SCRUTTON — Superintendent Physiotherapist, Newcomen Centre, Guy's Hospital, London SE1 9RT.

ANITA H. SLOMINSKI — Co-ordinator, Cerebral Palsy Treatment Center, Department of Orthopedics, Indiana University School of Medicine, Indianapolis.

THOMAS TILLEMANS — Professor, School of Education, Acadia University, Wolfville, Nova Scotia, Canada.

VACLAV VOJTA — Neurologist and Child Neurologist, Vice Director and Chairman of the Department of Physiotherapy of Kinderzentrum München, West Germany.

ROSEMARY WHITE — Registered Occupational Therapist, Specialist in Developmental Disabilities, Seattle, Washington.

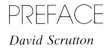

PREFACE

David Scrutton

This book is about cerebral palsy, defined by the Little Club in 1964 as 'a permanent, but not unchanging disorder of movement and posture due to a non-progressive defect or lesion of the brain in early life' (cited by Christensen and Melchior 1967). This definition is not universally agreed but it describes very well the area the book will be covering. Currently there is some discussion whether the term 'cerebral palsy' has outlived its usefulness and become too restrictive, but I find it a useful grouping for a variety of disorders which retain enough in common with each other, and sufficient differences from (say) late acquired or progressive disorders, to help in planning management.

The general interest in the habilitation of those having cerebral palsy is comparatively modern, but predates the sharp decline in the incidence of polio and tuberculosis. The concern, fostered by a few orthopaedic surgeons and physicians, was eagerly taken up by therapists, and the variety of approaches to treatment has been the cause of much—often heated—debate over the last forty years.

However, time has mellowed attitudes and more recently a subtle but significant change has occurred, probably set in motion by three factors. Firstly, the emergence of paediatricians with a greater interest in chronic handicap; secondly, a change in social attitude—an appreciation that those with severe handicap have lives to lead as well as disorders to be treated; and lastly, I consider that the therapists themselves have changed and become more relaxed in their approach to their patients and also towards themselves and their treatments. These changes have allowed an altogether less partisan and more open attitude to discussion.

It seemed to me that a book in which I described or interpreted different treatment approaches would be bound to reflect my own bias and be open to the criticism that I did not fully appreciate this or that treatment or viewpoint. So instead I asked those whose treatments bore the mark of individuality to write a chapter explaining their aims, rationale and what they do, and I am grateful to all the authors for their willing acceptance of certain editorial constraints. If they were unable to write a chapter themselves, they were asked to recommend an alternative author.

The list of authors and their subjects is not comprehensive, but it is representative of current practice. Even so, some readers will miss their favoured approach and perhaps they deserve a short explanation. There was one chapter which could have been written only by one person, who unfortunately was prevented from doing so by other commitments. In spite of being well known, two treatments were omitted because no one could be found with sufficient current experience to write an authoritative chapter. Some treatments were discounted because their aims were too limited to be seen as more than a technique which, although used for cerebral palsy, was not particularly relevant to it. A very few treatments were omitted because I considered them ethically unacceptable. None was excluded on the grounds of being 'ineffective': too little is known to make such judgements.

There are two additional chapters, and an introduction to the subject for those unfamiliar with the physical management of cerebral palsy. Chapter 4 is a summary of my own views on the management of these children; while the last chapter rounds off the book by putting physical treatment and management into a neurological context.

It is not the aim of this book to steer a course through this maze of (often conflicting) advice and come to a helpful conclusion, nor to teach how cerebral palsy should be treated. Rather, it is an attempt to present some of the factors which need consideration by those involved with cerebral palsy and to leave the reader with a wider appreciation of the many points of view.

REFERENCE

Christensen, E., Melchior, J. C. (1967) *Cerebral Palsy—a Clinical and Neuropathological Study. Clinics in Developmental Medicine, No. 25.* London: Spastics Society with Heinemann Medical. p. 1.

FOREWORD

Bruce Gans

When David Scrutton called to ask me to write the Foreword to this book I was both honored and perplexed. Honored to be considered for inclusion in such a notable project, but perplexed as to what I might say. The collective knowledge and experience of the various authors is exhaustive—what more could be said? But as I reviewed the manuscript, it became clear that there was still more to be said. There were hidden assumptions, attitudes and opinions that pervaded the text. They are worth stating explicitly.

Firstly, there is the underlying expression of care and concern for the plight of the physically disabled child. Not only do these authors care, they have tried to do something; and they have dedicated their lives to sharing their concern and knowledge with others. Secondly, they believe that without their care and intervention, children will not grow and develop to achieve their full motor capabilities. And thirdly, it is believed that the intervention must be early, consistent, and of long-term duration to be truly effective.

But why do so many and such highly divergent approaches exist? And why is there such controversy and apparent incompatibility between them? There are probably several answers to these questions. Common human experience teaches us that the greater the number of 'solutions' proposed for a problem, the more difficult and truly insoluble it probably is. Furthermore, the greater the need, the more that people feel compelled to do something, indeed anything, rather than merely to accept a condition as irremediable. This leads us back to fundamental principles. The child with brain damage cannot be expected to live up to the potential ordained for one with a normal brain structure. The learning (in this context, motor learning) that the child will achieve will be at a greater cost and need closer attention than otherwise. There is a price to be paid for that achievement.

Clearly there are elements of truth in the teachings of each of the approaches presented here. Equally, none is likely to be the one and only truth. We need to remember that in any therapeutic relationship there are two sides; the patient in need, and the therapist with skills to provide. An individual therapist is, in all likelihood, going to have greatest proficiency in one particular technique (that most believed and most practised). This means that the needs of the child, the skills of the therapist, and social, cultural, geographic, and financial factors will all contribute to the determination of what is the 'right' therapy for an individual child.

There is another perspective to the disabled child that we must keep in mind: that a child is usually connected to a parental unit. The needs of that child's family, as well as their capacities, must be considered in the determination of what is right. Families frequently place great faith and trust in the hands of those helping them to cope with the problems of their disabled child. With that faith and trust comes an even greater responsibility for the therapist not to make matters worse for the family than they already are. Guilt is a frequent factor in the psychology of parenting a cerebral-palsied child. When we establish therapeutic goals and objectives for a child we may be unintentionally setting up the family for further failures (particularly if their hidden objective is far greater than the stated explicit aim of treatment). A program that is too demanding of time and attention from family and friends may seriously stress an already fragile set of relationships within the family and local community; and such an intense focus on the motor disability may distract a family from focusing upon other aspects of a child's needs, and particularly may prevent effective long-term planning.

How, then, can you the reader learn from this book? Read it carefully, perhaps several times, and think about what you are reading. Put into perspective the techniques and philosophies presented with your own personal skills and environment. Match the needs of your children and their families with the best that you and those around you can provide. But always be sure that you are helping, rather than adding to the already overwhelming burden of living with cerebral palsy.

INTRODUCTION

David Scrutton

Treatment classification

How and, indeed, whether to treat cerebral palsy are questions which must trouble many paediatricians. Those who take the time to seek a policy they can apply to their patients have seldom been satisfied by what they have found on lifting the stone marked 'therapy'. Many therapists share this dissatisfaction. However, this situation is not surprising when one considers the number of variables within each so-called 'type' of cerebral palsy, the frequent additional handicaps, differing family attitudes and social circumstances and a host of other environmental factors such as the limitations imposed by the available medical and educational facilities. Doctors can choose to ignore these complexities simply by referring the child for 'therapy'; therapists cannot. Faced with the child and the parents' expectations, they have to do something. The different treatments are their responses to this challenge.

Therapists derive professional satisfaction from analysing a patient's problem into its treatable components and applying their treatment skills. In neuro-developmental disorders, however, such a straightforward approach is less appropriate, for the child being treated has to be seen both as he is and as the adult he will become. This can change both the aims and the means of treatment. How can the patient best be helped to maximise his potential as an adult? It is the response to this question that so often divides treatments from each other, and it is in their aims quite as much as in their treatment methods that treatments differ. It is also what makes them so difficult to compare. How can one compare 'successes' when the aims are different? One person's success is seen as a treatment failure by another.

As a start, treatment success could be defined by the functional result rather than a more clinically based assessment. Bleck (1979), for instance, grades walking ability as community walker, household walker, physiological walker (walking only in a physical therapy department) and non-walker, each category having a real-life meaning: the implication being that a treatment should result in a better grading. Of course this is not quite so, as the difference between only just achieving a grade and easily achieving it can be very real indeed, functionally and cosmetically; but the grading imparts a salutory message to the treater. However, the question I am considering goes beyond this. The motor disorder should not be treated simply because it is there, but only insofar as our intervention reduces the *over-all* handicap of the child and potential adult. Whatever the grading, whatever the skill, it may have little to do with succeeding as a person. Of course, the ability to walk and how one walks (say) is important, but so too is a reason for walking. To make walking worthwhile, the adult needs a reason for living which can be perceived as having the possibility of fulfilment and we must ensure that our intervention does not interfere too greatly with the development of intellect, drive, personality, communication and education.

It is in such a total context that treatment results must be judged and intervention be based. I agree that this is no easy task—but the problem is still there. If I appear to exaggerate, talk to the young adults with years of treatment and special schooling behind them.

There is, however, a rather more immediate obstacle to assessing treatment success: children develop. Changes (some advantageous, some not) will be occurring all the time whether we treat or not; and when one considers the multitude of variables which can influence the child from day to day it is hard to ascribe any change to one particular variable—therapy.

Therefore, without common diagnostic criteria, reliable prognosis, an obvious common goal and accurate assessment of treatment outcome, a wide variety of treatment approaches and techniques have evolved. Here are some criteria by which they might be classified.

Rationale

There are three foundations for rationale:

Mechanical: based on muscle power, joint range, line of gravity, base, mass, and postural stability. It naturally leads to treatments which influence these factors and is probably the most easily understood approach.

Neurological: treatments based on different aspects of neurology; peripheral, utilising exteroception and proprioception to facilitate or inhibit muscle action; and central, which by a variety of means and to differing degrees set out to influence the disorder or the effect of the disorder by changing, if not the structure, at least the function of the damaged central nervous system.

Educational: a viewpoint creating treatments in which intervention becomes more akin to 'education' than 'treatment'.

All treatments will have elements of each rationale, one of which will be prominent. The mechanical approach does not overlook that a knee is flexed from a neurological cause, but that straightening the knee is best done by treatment to the leg rather than the central nervous system. And so on. Furthermore different rationales do not always lead to different treatments, although their aims might be different.

Scope

Some treatments have quite specific and limited aims: methods of relaxing spastic muscles or increasing postural stability at a joint. Other treatments have a global approach to the child and almost take on the rôle of a philosophy of treatment. These latter approaches tend to encourage a way of thinking about the disorder from which the therapist can construct a 'solution' to any problem which arises in the course of treatment. Such an approach to cerebral palsy, with all its variations and complexities, can be useful and reassuring both to the therapist and the child's parents.

Who does the treatment

Some treatments require special skills and experience and although parents or care staff could be shown how to do them, they would be unlikely to be competent enough to make it worthwhile. Other treatments are specifically designed to be done by lay people, their effect being enhanced by constant application (which no therapist could achieve) rather than diminished through lack of expertise. Whilst it may be obvious that some of the specific treatment techniques may require special skills from the therapist, it may not be so apparent that this also applies to the lay treatments. The formulation of a treatment programme (however simple it might appear) and instruction of parents is not something that anyone can do without guidance or experience.

Primary aim
Some treatments aim for better patterns of movement, greater postural stability and increased joint range, in the expectation that these will automatically expand the child's movement opportunities and so increase function. Other treatments aim directly for function, considering that it is the abilities and attitudes engendered in the child which are of primary importance, and that treatments not so directed do not automatically lead to increased day-to-day competence and may impede other aspects of the child's development.

Age
The suitability of a treatment may depend on the child's age in two ways: a treatment may be inappropriate because it requires co-operation from the child which cannot be expected of the infant or the younger child, or methods of handling by the therapist which cannot easily be achieved if the child is too big. Equally, the rationale may be based on neuro-developmental considerations, relying on the 'plasticity' of the as yet uncommitted central nervous system, aiming to influence the development of new skills prior to or during their emergence. Thus some treatments are suitable only for particular ages or stages of development whilst others may be applicable throughout life.

As with any classification these categories cannot be comprehensive; other factors subdivide the treatments. However, I consider that these five allow a comparison of treatments which may be of particular help to readers not directly involved in treating cerebral-palsy children. So the best treatment for a child depends on (i) the particular child, (ii) his circumstances and (iii) the inclinations of the person treating. Rational judgements cannot be made because there is little if any evidence on the effects of these treatments. It is generally accepted that this lack of evidence is due mainly to the complexity of the condition and will not easily be overcome.

The uncertainty of very early diagnosis and imprecise prognosis dictates that alterations of outcome through treatment are most likely to be shown from trials involving large numbers. An incidence of approximately two per thousand livebirths makes this difficult and would involve multicentre trials requiring standardised diagnostic terminology (which is difficult*) and standardised treat-

---

*The most significant differences to treatment response in hypertonic cerebral palsy seem to be the subtle variations in spasticity and rigidity and the particular patterns of posture and movement. It is on these points that terminology is so weak and agreement non-existent.

ments (which for all but the simplest is nearly impossible). It seems likely that progress will be made first of all in two areas: assessing specific *techniques* applied to specific presenting signs secondary to cerebral palsy (*e.g.* prevention or correction of deformity) and the gradual introduction of more reliable prognostic tests.

Early treatment
In the meantime, whilst not decrying the need for treatment of older children or adults, most therapists favour early treatment and there is general agreement that the younger the child the greater the effect of the treatment. There are a number of reasons for this:

(1) Massive myelination is occurring. It is probably easier to form correct movement habits before incorrect ones are established.

(2) Most parents expect to devote a large proportion of their time to a baby during its first two years of life and so it is easier and more realistic to involve them in treatment.

(3) Treatment does not interfere with the education and social life of the child (but see Chapter 2).

(4) It is a time when parents need close contact with someone who understands their problems in a constructive manner, gives them something positive to do and can help them to find out about and to understand their child's emerging difficulties.

The cynical will suggest that it is easier to ameliorate (or even 'cure') a disorder which may not be present than one which is definitely present, and it must be admitted that there is probably a not inconsiderable proportion of normal-but-different babies treated 'successfully' in the age-group under three months. (Incidence figures might help to clarify this, but few treatment centres truly know of their liveborn catchment population.) However, this alone should not be allowed to prevent early treatment.

Physical therapy associated with orthopaedic surgery
It is not the purpose of this book to discuss the physical treatment associated with orthopaedic surgery, which is quite separate from a general discussion of therapy for cerebral-palsied children. Some clinicians look upon surgery as an alternative to physical treatment, as a sign of therapy failure or as a last resort. Nothing could be further from the truth: it is the treatment of choice in many situations and a worthwhile option in others; but essentially it is part of an over-all plan of physical management for the child. Indeed, in some clinics it is the orthopaedic surgeon who is primarily responsible for that plan.

Nevertheless, surgery is a discrete and dramatic event which may radically change a child's abilities, potential or day-to-day care. For a while the post-operative treatment may have to take priority over most other competing aims if the child is not to lose a unique locomotor opportunity. Time off from school may be needed for treatment or hospital visits for orthotics and modifications to wheelchairs *etc.* The child's posture may need to be strictly controlled during parts of the day and at night. All this can be disruptive, but it is justified by the long-term benefit. However, not all surgery needs to make such demands; and many children, after (say) heel cord lengthening, do just as well without physical therapy as with it. Post-operative management needs discussion with the parents and teachers pre-operatively so that they have a good understanding of what will be required of themselves and the child, and can make arrangements accordingly.

The actual post-operative treatment is well within the ability of any physical therapist, but there are certain typical problems that can arise and need to be recognised early, so it is a great advantage to have had experience with cerebral palsy. The treatment itself is straightforward: strengthening certain muscle actions, maintaining increased joint range, supporting unstable joints and improving static and dynamic posture. Clearly stated review dates are needed for the various aspects of treatment, so that the child can return to a more normal routine at the first opportunity.

When dealing with complex and ill-understood situations, it is simplicity and attention to detail which seem most often to meet with success; and I refer here to the surgery quite as much as the therapy.

REFERENCE

Bleck, E. E. (1979) *Orthopaedic Management of Cerebral Palsy. Saunders Monographs in Clinical Orthopaedics.* Philadelphia: W. B. Saunders.

1
THE NEURO-DEVELOPMENTAL TREATMENT

Karel and Berta Bobath

Aims

The aim of treatment for children with cerebral palsy or other conditions involving the upper motor neuron of the CNS, regardless of aetiology, is to lead them towards the greatest degree of independence possible, and so prepare them for as normal an adolescent and adult life as can be achieved. This is the aim of all schools of treatment. It involves establishing for the child a total management programme, in which specialised physiotherapy forms an essential part. By definition, cerebral palsy is due to damage or maldevelopment of the brain in earliest childhood, which interferes with the child's growth and maturation. Therefore, it involves the total development of the child—sensorimotor, physical, mental, emotional and social. Frequently the various associated sensory and perceptual losses are secondary to the physical handicap, which prevents him exploring himself; thus he does not develop a concept of his body—the so-called 'body percept' as does a normal child during the first 18 months, prior to orienting himself in space (Piaget 1977, Pularski 1979).

This lack of 'body percept' can be accentuated by the parents' inexperience and inability to deal with the handicap, and seems to us one of the main arguments for early recognition and management of cerebral palsy. It is just as important as the prevention of contractures and deformities, which are not present at birth but may develop later in childhood as the child makes use of abnormal patterns of movement in compensatory functional activity.

Rationale

Our treatment has developed gradually over the last 40 years. It is not a 'method', as it is neither rigid nor standardised. It takes into account that cerebral palsy and allied conditions comprise a group of symptoms in which there is great variety; therefore treatment has to be flexible and adapted to the many and varied needs of the individual child. No *standardised* set of exercises will be adequate to the needs of all children.

We believe that the handicap of cerebral-palsied children arises fundamentally from an interference with the development of normal postural control against gravity (Bobath 1980). The brain lesion results in the release of abnormal patterns of co-ordination, in association with various types of abnormality of postural tone and disordered reciprocal innervation. For instance, in the spastic child a group of phylogenetically more primitive patterns of posture against gravity appear and become dominant in a pathological form. They can cause spasticity, loss of mobility and disturbance of reciprocal innervation, with excessive fixation in typical abnormal patterns. Furthermore, there is exaggerated and abnormal co-

contraction of antagonistic muscle groups (especially proximally) or abnormal reciprocal 'tonic inhibition': for example, spastic flexors of the forearm inhibiting extension of the elbow. Commonly spasticity is regarded as a release phenomenon of the gamma-system (more rarely of the alpha-system) from higher control (Magoun and Rhines 1946, Matthews 1964, Granit 1968, Eccles 1972). It is usually tested by assessing the degree of resistance a muscle group offers to passive stretch. This localised testing for spasticity has guided therapy since the first description of this condition by Little in 1862 (reprinted 1958). However, it neglects the rather obvious observation that spasticity affects whole muscular systems in typical patterns; and it does not take into account the fact that spasticity is very changeable and increases with stimulation and effort.

In the dyskinetic athetoid groups of cerebral palsy we find a basically low tonus at rest, but it is unstable and fluctuates with stress and stimulation. Furthermore, the amplitude of this fluctuation varies in the individual patient. Abnormal reciprocal innervation shows itself in a lack of ability to make a graduated movement because of sudden and more or less total inhibition of the antagonists.

The term 'athetosis' was coined by Hammond (1871) and means no fixed posture. Athetoid children are unable to maintain stable postures because of lack of co-contraction. Similar problems of low tonus and disturbed reciprocal innervation can be seen in the ataxic child and in the 'dysequilibrium' syndrome described by Hagberg *et al.* (1972). This explains why athetosis is often combined with ataxia (Twitchell 1959, 1961).

Among the athetoid group, the dystonic type of cerebral palsy is demonstrated by intermittent spasms of varying strength and amplitude (Polani 1959). Abnormally low tone is also seen in the so-called 'floppy' infant (Dubowitz 1980). Such infants with cerebral palsy subsequently may develop athetosis or ataxia (Lesny 1979).

The changes in emphasis of treatment
Since we began our treatment in 1943 we have been learning constantly, and experience has taught us to change our approach and our emphasis on certain aspects of the treatment. However, the basic concept has not changed. Throughout we have been guided by the child's reactions to our handling, and in this way we have improved our knowledge and tried to avoid repeating mistakes. We have learned to test the value of a particular technique by the child's response to it, and have developed an approach based on the close interplay between child and therapists.

We used to describe the motor patterns of the hypertonic child, both spastic and dystonic, in terms of the release of the few tonic reflexes described, among others, by Magnus (1926), Rademaker (1935) and Byers (1938). To these belong the tonic neck and tonic labyrinthine reflexes and the positive supporting reactions (Bobath 1971). We grossly overrated these reflexes in explaining the abnormal patterns of the hypertonic child. These reflexes have been studied in experimental animals, and while they have a certain influence and can be seen more clearly in some severe types of cerebral palsy, they are inadequate to account for the varied abnormal patterns of most hypertonic children. Even in severe cases they are inconstant, depending on the degrees of excitation and effort when testing. We no longer include them in our assessment of children.

The most important tonic reflex activities seen in spastic children are the so-called 'associated reactions' (Walshe 1923). They have been defined as general tonic reflexes acting from one part of the body on the rest of the affected parts, and it must be kept in mind that any voluntary movement performed with effort when treating one part of the body increases spasticity in another affected part. In the hypertonic child, therefore, they contribute to the development of contractures and deformities because they accentuate the patterns of spasticity.

Over the years we have been influenced by and have learned from other workers in the field. For example, we have learned from Knott (1952), Kabat and Knott (1953) and Knott and Voss (1973), and have recognised the importance of proprioceptive stimulation to build up tonus in patients with low and unstable postural tone. From Rood (1954) and Goff (1969, 1972) we have learned the value of tactile stimulation to obtain movements, especially of hands, feet, mouth and tongue. We have learned most, however, from Petö (Cotton and Parnwell 1967, Clarke and Evans 1973) who, like us, saw that the problem for these children was inco-ordination of function, and this helped us better to prepare athetoid children for everyday life. We are still learning from our mistakes and omissions.

We found that our early 'reflex-inhibiting postures' reduced spasticity by modifying its patterns. However, the child was passively positioned and the postures controlled the whole child, preventing any movement, so there was no carry-over into movement and function. We then found a way of using 'key points of control' from which patterns of abnormal activity could be inhibited, while at the same time facilitating normal movements. The child then could move actively where not actually held, and the quality of movements could be guided and controlled from key points. In this way we could facilitate whole sequences of active movements and prevent deterioration by the return of hypertonus.

For a while our treatment concentrated too much upon the facilitation of the automatic righting reactions; we had hoped that by giving the child the normal background of movements—facilitating Schaltenbrand's 'principal motility'—the child would spontaneously translate it into functional and voluntary movements. This worked well with very young babies, but when it came to sitting and the use of hands, standing and walking—activities which all require balance—we found it inadequate. We saw that the child who lacked balance was afraid of falling when he had to move or be moved against gravity and that hypertonus then increased again, with deterioration of movements. The need to obtain good balance reactions, and the detrimental effect on movement when they are insufficient or absent, is still one of our greatest problems.

We learned that it was necessary to reduce our control gradually, handing it over increasingly and systematically to the child, and so allow him control of his own movement, especially of balance. We had to alternate techniques of facilitiation and inhibition when hypertonus interfered at certain stages of a movement, and this led to improved interaction between therapist and child. A further logical step was to make a careful study of the development of movement as it occurs in normal babies. However, we soon found that it was not enough—indeed it was wrong—to try to follow the normal developmental sequence too closely. We had made the child rigidly go through the stage of rolling over, before going on to sitting, side-sitting, kneeling, kneel-standing, half-kneeling, crawling and then finally standing; one stage after the other. But that sequence is not followed faithfully by normal children. Contrary to the impression that could be gained from charts of development such as Gesell (1947), Griffiths (1954) and Illingworth (1960), development often does not proceed in a definite sequence, in which 'milestones' follow each other. Obviously these charts can give only isolated activities which are characteristic of certain chronological ages, but they cannot take into account the wide variation in age of attainment. They are of use in detecting retarded or arrested development, but they are unreliable for early diagnosis of the child with cerebral palsy, and of even less use in assessment and planning of treatment. Normal children develop many activities simultaneously, which reinforce each other to culminate in a 'milestone'. Also it is well known that development may come to a temporary halt in one sphere, or even regress, while the child pushes ahead in another sphere. Instead of a definite sequential pattern, it seems that the baby develops some basic motor patterns of co-ordination which at any one stage enables performance of a number of different activities (Bobath and Bobath 1970).

The last stage of the development of our treatment was the recognition of the fact that the treatment was not carried over into activities of daily life, as we had expected it would be. Both parents and children regarded the treatment as a set of exercises, remote from functional use at home. We saw, for example, that it did very little for prehension and manipulation. It became obvious that a more direct transition of treatment was needed to make it useful in the home and in performing functional skills. This is where we are now; we are still learning and (we hope) improving. Treatment now incorporates systematic preparation for specific functions, and we realise the need for thorough analysis of each task we try to prepare the child to perform. We relate this analysis to the assessment of the needs of the individual child, finding out what interferes with or what is missing from each part of that task. We aim at treating the children in 'functional situations', *i.e.* those in which they live at home or at school, to ensure that the tasks are carried over into daily life. As far as possible we use the same furniture they are used to; we treat them while they are dressed or undressed; when being fed or feeding themselves. Treatment can be done while the child sits on a tricycle, in his pram or on his pot. All this, of course, goes side by side with more specific treatment for his basic problems or abnormal tonus and qualities of motor patterns.

Treatment
The treatment is done by 'handling' the child; he guides us and we guide him by means of constant feedback. We guide the motor output by our handling to make the child's reactions as normal as possible during treatment. In this way he can

experience by repetition and establish new and more normal sensorimotor patterns.

Abnormal patterns of posture and movement are closely related to abnormal tonus (Bernstein 1967), just as normal patterns are to normal tonus. Therefore normal movements obtained during treatment will normalise tonus. With a hypertonic child we counteract (inhibit) the abnormal patterns of released postural reflex activity, and at the same time facilitate normal reactions by special techniques of handling. In this way we aim at obtaining and guiding his active movements of postural adjustment to our handling. Facilitation means 'making easy', but in treatment it also means 'making possible' and making it necessary for a movement to happen (Bobath and Bobath 1964, Bryce 1972).

We avoid encouraging strong voluntary effort from a spastic child because it increases spasticity and produces associated reactions. The desired movement can be elicited by using less voluntary and more automatic movements, for instance in play. With athetoid children we have to be careful not to increase spasms and involuntary movements, but we can enlist their voluntary control of the movements. With ataxic children we try to avoid the occurrence of intention tremor. Therefore we have to grade motivation, increasing it carefully, and not use indiscriminate sensory stimulation. We have to keep in mind that the child with cerebral palsy is unable to react normally, even to normal sensory input; he can only react with his abnormal output, the only type the damaged brain puts at his disposal. The problem therefore is not so much one of modification of input, but of influence and control of the output. This is done by the natural stimulation of handling and play, stopping the motor response to the stimulation from flowing into abnormal patterns of posture and movement. The situation is different for children with minimal cerebral palsy or with motor retardation who have primitive but normal co-ordinated motor activity; for them sensory stimulation is of prime importance (Ayres 1966, 1972).

We do not 'correct' the postures of cerebral-palsied children because their abnormal co-ordination means that correction of one part of the body merely transfers the abnormal pattern to another part. We also do not 'teach' these children movements, since they can only do them abnormally; instead we make more normal movements possible during treatment. Cerebral palsy is a sensorimotor problem. We do not learn movements but the sensation of movements, so we help the child to experience the sensation of more normal movements and of movements he has not done before. The child with cerebral palsy has memories only of abnormal movements, since he has had no experience of others, and many essential postures and movements are missing altogether. These children need to experience normal movements during treatment and, by training the parents, to be able to carry them over into life at home.

When making a treatment plan we should consider that many motor activities develop simultaneously, and that in fact they overlap with prehension and manipulation. For instance, around the seventh month the normal baby can roll over, creep on his abdomen along the floor, sit and balance with arm support and stand supported. Around nine months he can sit up from prone by himself and does not need his arms for support when sitting. He can also crawl on all fours, or on his hands and feet, pull himself to stand and walk around holding on to furniture. However, these ages are only approximate and there is wide individual variation. Achievement of motor activities is culturally determined and varies with nursing care and habit. Some children pull themselves to stand before they sit unsupported, some do not crawl on all fours, but immediately get onto hands and feet, or shuffle on their bottoms about the floor (Robson and Mac Keith 1971). Head control when pulled to sit is delayed in children who are nursed mainly in the prone position. It is also delayed in prone when the child has been nursed mainly in sitting and supine positions.

Treatment should not attempt to follow the sequence of development described, regardless of the age and physical condition of the individual child. Rather, it should be decided what each child needs most urgently at any one stage or age, and what is absolutely necessary for him in preparation for future functional skills, or for improving the skills he has but performs abnormally. We should know which motor patterns, essential for specific function, are missing and should be developed. But we also have to counteract abnormal patterns which prevent proper function. There is no time to waste on unspecific, general, developmental treatment, for we cannot expect that such treatment will automatically carry over into functional skills later on.

Treatment should not try to perfect one specific activity. Valuable time would be lost, and as the child with cerebral palsy is unable to perform the movement with normal co-ordination—even with the best of treatment—practice and repetition of these movements over long periods will perpetuate and reinforce the abnormal pattern instead of improving it. Even normal children never perfect one activity before going on to the next; in fact it is by attempting a more difficult task that they perfect the previous activity. For example, he already stands when he learns to balance in sitting, and when he starts to walk holding onto the furniture he is still perfecting crawling on all fours. For this reason we should not single out and try to perfect specific milestones, *i.e.* work for long periods on sitting, kneeling and crawling. For treatment, we should choose the movements which belong together at any developmental level. Instead of concentrating solely on sitting or creeping, we should combine rolling with sitting up from prone, and sitting with balance and arm support as well as with the use of hands for reaching out and for play, or to help with dressing. We should combine prone lying with creeping on the abdomen, or combine sitting with kneeling and standing up. The aim should be to obtain dynamic sequences of movements rather than more or less static abilities.

We also should keep in mind what Milani-Comparetti called the 'competition of patterns', which happens even in the normal child when he tries to do something new and more difficult. Established and well co-ordinated movements may disappear or deteriorate for a short time, until the new skill has become easy and automatic. These 'regressive' patterns may be seen, for example, when normal babies first try to pull themselves up to stand, or to use their hands for fine manipulation, but they are not abnormal. Grady *et al.* (1981) has called these clumsy patterns 'primitive abnormal'. The competition of patterns is a great danger in treatment if one concentrates for a long period on one activity. The child with cerebral palsy may take much longer than the normal child to acquire a new movement, and that movement pattern then becomes dominant. An example of this is a child who continues crawling on all fours and cannot progress to standing and walking. For children with spastic diplegia and quadriplegia there is the additional danger of developing flexor contractures at hips and knees. Therefore our knowledge of the overlap of motor function in normal child development should lead us to rely on the combination of related activities and sequences of movement.

Techniques of treatment
Techniques of treatment are important, but are only tools, and should not be held responsible for obtaining results. Only those that answer the special needs of the individual child at a particular age and stage of treatment should be selected. Special training and experience should enable us to assess what *might* work in a particular case. No technique is suitable for all children, and there is no reason to think that because a technique has been successful with one child it will also improve another child, even if the problem is similar. The therapist's approach should be that it *may* work, and if it does not—the criterion being the response of the child—it should be changed or discarded. It is most important to give the child a chance and the time to react, to wait for the response, then to evaluate its quality and to adjust one's treatment to it. Above all, the therapist must know *how* to use techniques and only use those which give an immediate change for the better under her hands, *i.e.* within one treatment session. Eclectic treatment, using a mixture of treatment techniques derived from various schools of thought which see the child's problems from different viewpoints, cannot result in a cohesive treatment programme (Bobath 1967, Levitt 1977).

A systematic and adequate treatment plan requires the thorough assessment of each child, otherwise valuable time can be lost by doing things which are unimportant and not dealing with the main problems, or by treatment which is too easy or too difficult for the child. We have to find out the causes of his difficulties and how his various problems—*e.g.* physical, emotional, social, perceptual—are interrelated. We want to know *why* the child cannot perform a certain movement or skill, or why he does it abnormally. We want to know what interferes with his movements, and which movement patterns of a specific skill he has missed in his development. This knowledge gives us information for preparing him to attain the skills expected for his chronological age. Assessment and treatment not only help us to plan further treatment, but also make it possible to compare progress. However, in addition to the initial assessment, we also assess and re-assess the child at all times during treatment by watching his reactions to it.

How often to treat, and whether to treat or merely to train parents in home management, depends on the individual child and his physical condition. Often parental training and guidance is sufficient with a retarded child who has no physical problems. Obviously the frequency of treatment sessions depends on the severity of the condition and on the need to prevent or ameliorate contractures.

Advantages and problems of very early treatment
There are many reasons why cerebral-palsied children benefit more from early treatment than from treatment given at a later age (Bobath 1967). Early treatment, at around three to four months of age, is important because of the great adaptability and plasticity of the infantile brain. During the first 18 months of a child's life there is great and speedy development, and at no other stage of growth does the child learn so quickly. It is a time in which not only is there the highest potential for learning, but also for adjustment to cerebral palsy.

Learning to move is entirely dependent on sensory experience. The normal child changes and modifies his inborn sensorimotor patterns, and adapts them to more complex functions such as prehension and walking. We know from recent studies with ultrasonic photography (Nilsson *et al.* 1973) and cine film (Milani-Comparetti 1981, Ianniruberto and Tajani 1981), and from the observations of Burns and Bullock (1980), that the baby *in utero* already experiences a wealth of beautifully co-ordinated movements, long before birth. From birth onward he uses and adapts the same movements in response to the increasing demands of extra-uterine life, for control against gravity, self-help and skills. If sensorimotor experience is abnormal from the beginning (as with a cerebral-palsied child) he will be able to make use only of his abnormal motor patterns. If not too severely affected, the intelligent child adapts these abnormal patterns to functional use, and so perpetuates and reinforces them.

In most cases very early treatment will give quicker and better results because the baby does not yet show much abnormality and therefore has little experience of abnormal movements. Furthermore, because treatment and handling are easier for the mother and therapist, the mother can more easily be instructed and trained in the best way of handling her baby. Usually she is already handling the baby all day long, dressing, carrying, feeding, washing, *etc.* Her involvement in management and treatment helps in establishing a good mother-child relationship and also gives her support and encouragement. It helps to prevent over-protection, as well as rejection. In fact, advice and training of the mother enables her to obtain the most normal active movements of the baby in response to her handling (Finnie 1974). She will learn to avoid abrupt handling, which can produce fear and discomfort in the infant and undue stretch of spastic muscles.

A problem in very early treatment is that often it is impossible to diagnose cerebral palsy under the age of four months, and even under six to eight months in slightly affected cases with 'soft neurological signs' (Ingram 1964). Initially the majority of cerebral-palsied babies do not show definite signs of abnormality, but mainly those of retardation (Ellenberg and Nelson 1981). If early diagnosis of cerebral palsy is extremely difficult, diagnosis of the type of cerebral palsy is even more so. We do not know whether the child will turn out to be spastic, athetoid, ataxic or to have a mixed condition. It is uncertain whether a child will have quadriplegia, diplegia, hemiplegia or paraplegia. Tonus may appear to be normal, but more often is too low. Only a very few children are too stiff to move at birth; some may recover spontaneously, others may remain severely and globally affected. In less severe cases, signs of spasticity, athetosis or ataxia usually are not seen until the child responds to environmental stimulation and tries to move against gravity.

In the majority of cases there is an abnormal birth history (Illingworth 1960), such as prematurity, anoxia, or asphyxia requiring intubation, oxygen and intensive care. These are the babies at risk, who will need careful follow-up. Recently premature babies have been 'treated' while still in the incubator, which may be of great value if the therapist becomes involved in the teaching of nurses and mothers in how to position and handle such babies.

Treatment should be started only when signs of abnormal tonus and movement patterns are seen. In most babies this happens after a 'silent' period, during which no treatment is necessary; but if suspicious signs develop, the mother must be advised and trained in the management of the baby at home.

The few babies who show definite signs of abnormality soon after birth, which do not clear up, are no problem as far as diagnosis is concerned. They will need treatment immediately, but unfortunately they are usually severe cases with a poor prognosis, despite early treatment. More mildly affected at-risk babies may develop quite normally, though some workers have found a degree of learning disability and clumsy motor activity at school-age (*e.g.* Köng 1972, Touwen 1979). Illingworth called this syndrome 'minimal cerebral dysfunction'.

The difficulties in early diagnosis and evaluation of treatment are compounded by the awareness that early abnormal signs may clear up spontaneously and without treatment (Illingworth 1971, Haidvogl and Tauffkirchen 1979). There are also many deviations from the so-called 'normal' which can be seen in perfectly normal babies and are part and parcel of normal development (Touwen 1976, 1978; Flehmig 1979; Bierman-van Eendenburg *et al.* 1981).

It is our conviction that no particular treatment of babies at risk can be proven more efficient than another. Nowadays, despite the difficulty of very early diagnosis, many at-risk babies are being 'preventively' treated and 'cured'. The difficulty in making an early diagnosis and, even more, in assessing the results of early treatment is borne out by a statistical evaluation of Vojta (1981). He states that out of 207 babies diagnosed and treated between one week and four months of age, 199 (96 per cent) were discharged with normal motor and mental activity. However, he goes on to say that it is possible that about half of these babies—diagnosed as 'symptomatic babies at risk'—may have been treated unnecessarily.

As mentioned earlier, it is not possible to recognise suspected cases of cerebral palsy with any certainty before four months of age. Ellenberg and Nelson (1981) made a study of more than 32,000 children examined at four months after birth, and re-examined at the age of seven years, to determine the presence of cerebral palsy. They found: 'of the children considered to be normal, one in a thousand had cerebral palsy at the age of seven years, compared with one in a hundred of those thought to be suspect. Of the children who had been definitely neurologically abnormal at four months, one in seven had disabling cerebral palsy by early school-age'.

Whether to tell the parents if there is a suspicion of cerebral palsy is a very difficult problem. If early on, *i.e.* before the end of the fourth month, when there may be signs of motor retardation and some mixed but uncertain pathology, the paediatrician is justified in avoiding distress to the parents (Egan *et al.* 1969). However, the child should be seen again regularly at short intervals, keeping in mind that at no other time is development as fast and changes as great as in the first 10 months. If the baby is responding well to the handling which the therapist recommends, it is safe to continue surveillance at increasingly longer intervals. However, treatment should be started as soon as pathology becomes more obvious.

Early changes in the child's condition and uncertainty about diagnosis also present difficulties in treatment. Some slightly affected babies will become normal or be only minimally affected, while others who seem to be slightly affected will turn out to be severe and need long-term treatment. Therefore we withhold prediction of outcome: we begin treatment, but watch carefully for changes for better or worse, and re-assess the infant frequently.

Another problem with early treatment is the need to stimulate and activate the child, without increasing the abnormal signs. Such abnormal signs occur when the child is encouraged and tries to function without the normal complement of movement patterns. Therefore the therapist has to be able to look ahead and to know what may happen. The natural history of events varies in different types of cerebral palsy (Bobath and Bobath 1957), so the therapist has to detect the first signs of future abnormal patterns and activities, and counteract them before they become established. Treatment frequently has to be changed and adjusted to the changes observed in the child's development and when he improves or deteriorates. It is a mistake to continue for months with the same treatment programme and techniques, hoping that one day they will give the expected results.

We should not think that we can *cure* cerebral palsy, even if the child is treated very early, or that we can change all cases to only 'minimal' cerebral palsy. However, if treatment is started before abnormal patterns of movement have become established, it can help the child to organise his potential abilities in what for him is the most normal way.

Parent training
Training and guiding the parents in home management is of the greatest importance. They should be regarded as members of the team of therapists, since the child is actually with the therapist for only a limited time and spends most of his time at home. Parent training is essential not only with babies, but also with older children. No amount of treatment can be effective unless the progress the child makes during treatment is carried over into everyday life and activities. Everyone concerned with the child's treatment and management should work closely together and have the same understanding of what is being done in treatment, and its aim.

In our centre we have the mothers, and sometimes the fathers, with us when we treat their children, and we explain what we are doing and why we are doing it. We do not give them lists of exercises, but practise with them so that they learn how to continue some of the treatment at home, and how to handle the child in order to help him with his own movements during the day. We want to help the parents understand why their child cannot perform certain movements, and why some movements are done abnormally and with great effort. Together with the parents, we observe the child to find out what interferes with his movement. Parent training takes time, and it is necessary that there be good contact and communication between therapist and parents (Bobath and Finnie 1970).

REFERENCES

Ayres, A. J. (1966) 'Interrelationships among perceptual-motor functions in children.' *American Journal of Occupational Therapy,* **20,** 68–71.
—— (1972) *Sensory Integration and Learning Disorders.* Los Angeles: Western Psychological Servives. pp. 113–129.
Bierman-van Eendenburg, M. E. C., Jurgens-van der Zee, A. A., Olinga, A. A., Huisjes, H. H., Touwen, B. C. L. (1981) 'Predictive value of neonatal neurological exmination: a follow-up study at 18 months.' *Developmental Medicine and Child Neurology,* **23,** 296–305.
Bernstein, N. (1967) *The Co-ordination and Regulation of Movements.* Oxford: Pergamon.
Bobath, B. (1967) 'The very early treatment of cerebral palsy.' *Developmental Medicine and Child Neurology,* **9,** 373–390.
—— (1971) 'Motor development: its effect on general development and application to the treatment of cerebral palsy.' *Physiotherapy,* **57,** 526–532.
—— Bobath, K. (1970) 'The problem of spasticity in the treatment of patients with lesions of the upper motor neuron. *In: Proceedings of the Sixth International Congress of the World Federation for Physical Therapists.* Amsterdam: Assen van Gorcum, pp. 456–464.
—— —— (1975) *Motor Development in the Different Types of Cerebral Palsy.* London: Heinemann Medical.
—— Finnie, N. R. (1970) 'Problems of communication between parents and staff in the treatment and management of children with cerebral palsy.' *Developmental Medicine and Child Neurology,* **12,** 629–635.
Bobath, K. (1980) *A Neurophysiological Basis for the Treatment of Cerebral Palsy. Clinics in Developmental Medicine No. 75.* London: S.I.M.P. with Heinemann Medical; Philadelphia: Lippincott.
—— Bobath, B. (1964) 'The facilitation of normal postural reactions and movements in the treatment of cerebral palsy.' *Physiotherapy,* **50,** 246–262.
Bryce, J. (1972) 'Facilitation of movement—Bobath approach.' *Physiotherapy,* **58,** 403–407.
Burns, Y. R., Bullock, M. I. (1980) 'Sensory and motor development of preterm babies.' *Australian Journal of Physiotherapy,* **26,** 229–243.
Byers, K. (1938) 'Tonic neck reflexes in children considered from a prognostic standpoint.' *American Journal of Diseases of Children,* **55,** 696–742.
Clarke, J. Evans, E. (1973) 'Rhythmical intention as a method of treatment for the cerebral palsied patients.' *Australian Journal of Physiotherapy,* **19,** 57–64.
Cotton, E., Parnwell, M. (1967) 'From Hungary: the Petö method.' *Special Education,* **56,** 7.
Dubowitz, V. (1980) *The Floppy Infant, 2nd Edn. Clinics in Developmental Medicine No. 76.* London: S.I.M.P. with Heinemann Medical; Philadelphia: Lippincott.
Eccles, J. C. (1972) *The Understanding of the Brain.* New York: McGraw-Hill.
Egan, D. F., Illingworth, R. S., Mac Keith, R. C. (1969) *Developmental Screening 0–5 Years. Clinics in Developmental Medicine No. 30.* London: S.I.M.P. with Heinemann Medical; Philadelphia: Lippincott.
Ellenberg, J. H., Nelson, K. B. (1981) 'Early recognition of infants at high risk for cerebral palsy: examination at age four months.' *Developmental Medicine and Child Neurology,* **23,** 705–716.
Finnie, N. R. (1974) *Handling the Cerebral Palsied Child at Home, 2nd Edn.* London: Heinemann Medical.
Flehmig, I. (1979) *Normale Entwicklung des Säuglings und ihre Abweichungen.* Stuttgart: Thieme.
Gesell, A. (1947) *Developmental Diagnosis, 2nd Edn.* New York: Harper.
Goff, B. (1969) 'Appropriate afferent stimulation.' *Physiotherapy,* **55,** 9–17.
—— (1972) 'The application of recent advances in neurophysiology to Miss M. Rood's concept of neuromuscular facilitation.' *Physiotherapy,* **58,** 409–415.
Grady, M., Gilfoyle, E., Moore, J. C. (1981) *Children Adapt.* Thorofare, N.J.: Charles B. Slack.

Granit, R. (1968) 'The functional role of the muscle spindle's primary end organs'. *Proceedings of the Royal Society of Medicine*, **61**, 69–78.

Griffiths, R. (1954) *The Abilities of Babies*. London: University of London Press.

Hagberg, B., Sanner, G., Steen, M. (1972) 'The dysequilibrium syndrome in cerebral palsy.' *Acta Paediatrica Scandinavica*, **61**, Suppl. 226.

Haidvogl, M., Tauffkirchen, E. (1979) 'Distinction between cerebral palsy and normal variation of motor development in infancy.' *Wiener Medizinische Wochenschrift*, **129**, 37–41.

Hammond, W. A. (1871) 'On athetosis.' *Medical Times (New York)*, **2**, 747.

Ianniruberto, A., Tajani, E. (1981) 'Ultrasonographic study of fetal movements.' *Seminars in Perinatology*, **5**, 175–181.

Illingworth, R. S. (1960) *The Development of the Infant and Young Child, Normal and Abnormal*. Edinburgh: E. and S. Livingstone.

—— (1971) 'Die Dianose der Zerebralparese im ersten Lebensjahr.' *In:* Matthias, H. H., Bruester, H. T., Zimmermann, H. (Eds.) *Spastisch Gelähmte Kinder*. Stuttgart: Thieme.

Ingram, T. T. S. (1964) *Paediatric Aspects of Cerebral Palsy*. Edinburgh: E. & S. Livingstone.

Kabat, H., Knott, M. (1953) 'Proprioceptive facilitation in the restoration techniques for treatment of paralysis.' *Physical Therapy Review*, **33**, 53–64.

Knott, M. (1952) 'Specialized neuromuscular technics in the treatment of cerebral palsy.' *Physical Therapy Review*, **32**, 73–75.

—— Voss, D. (1974) *Proprioceptive Neuromuscular Facilitation, 2nd Edn*. New York: Harper & Row.

Köng, E. (1972) 'Früherfassung zerebraler Bewegungsstörungen.' *Pädiatrische Fortbildung, Praxis*, **33**, 1–14.

Lesny, I. (1979) 'Follow-up study of hypotonic forms of cerebral palsy.' *Brain and Development*, **1**, 81–90.

Levitt, S. (1977) *Treatment of Cerebral Palsy and Motor Delay*. Oxford: Blackwell.

Little, W. J. (1862) 'On the influence of abnormal parturition, difficult labours, premature birth, and asphyxia neonatorum, on the mental and physical condition of the child, especially in relation to deformities.' *Transactions of the Obstetrical Society of London*, **3**, 293 (*Reprinted in: Cerebral Palsy Bulletin*, 1958, **1**, 5–36.)

Magnus, R. (1926) 'Some results of studies of the physiology of posture.' *Lancet*, **2**, 531–535, 585.

Magoun, H. W., Rhines, R. (1946) 'Inhibitory mechanisms in bulbar reticular formation.' *Journal of Neurophysiology*, **9**, 165–171.

Matthews, P. B. C. (1964) 'Muscle spindles and their motor control.' *Physiological Review*, **44**, 219–288.

Milani-Comparetti, A. (1981) 'The neurologic and clinical implications of studies of fetal motor behaviour.' *Seminars on Perinatology*, **5**, 183–189.

Nilsson, L., Ingelman-Sundberg, A., Wirsén, C. (1973) *The Everyday Miracle: a Child is Born, 2nd Edn*. London: Allen Lane.

Piaget, J. (1977) *The Origins of Intelligence in the Child*. London: Penguin Educational.

Polani, P. E. (1959) 'The natural clinical history of choreo-athetoid cerebral palsy.' *Guy's Hospital Reports*, **108**, 32–45.

Pularski, M. A. S. (1979) *Your Baby's Mind and How it Grows*. London: Cassell.

Rademaker, G. G. J. (1935) *Réactions Labyrinthiques et Equilibre l'Ataxie Labyrinthique*. Paris: Masson.

Robson, P., Mac Keith, R. C. (1971) 'Shufflers with spastic diplegic cerebral palsy: a confusing clinical picture.' *Developmental Medicine and Child Neurology*, **13**, 651–659.

Rood, M. (1954) 'Neurophysiological reactions as a basis for physical therapy.' *Physical Therapy Review*, **34**, 444–448.

Touwen, B. (1976) *Neurological Development in Infancy. Clinics in Developmental Medicine No. 58*. London: S.I.M.P. with Heinemann Medical; Philadelphia: Lippincott.

—— (1978) 'Variability and stereotypy in normal and deviant development.' *In:* Apley, J. (Ed.) *Care of the Handicapped Child. Clinics in Developmental Medicine No. 67*. London: S.I.M.P. with Hienemann Medical; Philadelphia: Lippincott.

—— (1979) *The Examination of the Child with Minor Neurological Dysfunction, 2nd Edn. Clinics in Developmental Medicine No. 71*. London: S.I.M.P. with Heinemann Medical: Philadelphia: Lippincott.

Twitchell, T. E. (1959) 'On the motor deficit in congenital bilateral athetosis.' *Journal of Nervous and Mental Disease*, **129**, 105–132.

—— (1961) 'The nature of the motor deficit in double athetosis.' *Archives of Physical Medicine and Rehabilitation*, **42**, 63–67.

17

Vojta, V. (1981) *Die zerebralen Bewegungsstörungen im Säuglingsalter, Früdiagnose und Frütherapie,* *3rd Edn.* Stuttgart: F. Enke. pp. 183–189.
Walshe, F. M. R. (1923) 'On certain tonic or postural reflexes in adult hemiplegia, with special reference to associated and so-called associated movements.' *Brain,* **46,** 1–37.

FURTHER READING

André-Thomas, Chesni, Y., Saint-Anne Dargassies, S. (1960) *The Neurological Examination of the Infant. Little Club Clinics in Developmental Medicine No. 1.* London: National Spastics Society.
Bax, M., Mac Keith, R. (1963) *Minimal Cerebral Dysfunction. Little Club Clinics in Developmental Medicine No. 10.* London: National Spastics Society with Heinemann Medical.
Casaer, P. (1979) *Postural Behaviour in Newborn Infants. Clinics in Developmental Medicine No. 72.* London: S.I.M.P. with Heinemann Medical; Philadelphia: Lippincott.
Illingworth, R. S. (1962) *An Introduction to Developmental Assessment in the First Year. Little Club Clinics in Developmental Medicine No. 3.* London: National Spastics Society.
Peiper, A. (1963) *Cerebral Function in Infancy and Childhood.* New York: Consultants Bureau; London: Pitman Medical.
Prechtl, H. F. R. (1977) *The Neurological Examination of the Full-term Newborn Infant, 2nd Edn. Clinics in Developmental Medicine No. 63.* London: S.I.M.P. with Heinemann Medical; Philadelphia: Lippincott.

2
CONDUCTIVE EDUCATION

Maria Hari and Thomas Tillemans

Introduction

For a proper understanding of Conductive Education (CE) the following may prove useful:

(1) The term CE is difficult to understand. It means education as organised by 'conductors'. The conductor is a generalist, licensed after four years of professional college-level training, who combines in her function what medicine, education, physio- and logo-therapy and psychology have to offer to the education of physcially handicapped children. CE is also 'conducive' to a desired goal. The conductor, like the person in front of the orchestra, is responsible for the total effect obtained through careful orchestration of the contributions made by the individual musicians, each one of whom remains responsible for his own playing. CE is a systematic approach, a practice supported by theories, now used in the education of the physically handicapped, but potentially also applicable to other chronic conditions. The child is actively engaged in his own learning. CE uses materials, few in number, but numerous in their applications. It aims at the maximum integration of the physically handicapped. During his waking hours the child will be surrounded by persons who have received or are receiving the same training at the Conductor's College, situated in the Institute for the Motor Disabled, Budapest.

(2) The Institute has as its motto: 'Not because, but in order to'. It is future- or goal-oriented, not focusing on the past or on the aetiology of the problem.

(3) Positive expectations on the part of the parents and conductors are important, but so also are the child's body image, his self-concept and perception of his environment.

(4) Motivation, when it is a general alertness, has an organic or neuropsychological basis, being related to the function of the reticular formation. The child's motivation is also influenced by the presence in his group of healthy examples with whom to identify. There is also specific motivation which is related to one subject area or narrow field of talented performance.

(5) A dysfunction is not a property of the child, but the product of the interaction between himself, or the way he is, and his environment, or the way he is perceived.

(6) Positive comments will reward the child when he demonstrates behaviour directed towards the relevant goal. Unwanted or inappropriate behaviour is not extinguished through negative comments, but by the suggestion of a different activity.

(7) Neither the College nor the Institute supports a 'cookbook' approach, in which conductors are expected to look up standard recipes for rapidly categorised problems.

(8) In 'rhythmic intention', the conductor employs the child's inner language to voice directions to himself, which is considered more effective than when the conductor continuously verbalises the directions. It also serves to involve the child in his own education.

(9) Children with cerebral palsy have a learning disorder, which affects not only their motor skills, but also the intake and elaboration of information, their expressive functions, and the feedback system, separately or together.

(10) Fragmentation of the child, as a result of each member of the multidisciplinary team concentrating on only one aspect of the child, is avoided by making the conductor the contact person for the supportive specialised services.

(11) The Institute stresses learning rather than treatment.

(12) It combines the concepts of task-analysis and that of the underlying abilities.

(13) Conductors aim at maximum independence: they seek to avoid holding the child or supporting him. They *will* assist when failure would otherwise be inevitable. Credit for accomplishment, however, should go to the child, not the conductor.

(14) The conductor has a great deal of autonomy. She can select the methods she considers to be most suitable for the child in her charge. Outsiders cannot prescribe to her, but she is prepared to discuss her approach with them.

Aims

The primary aim of Conductive Education is to stimulate a developmental process which would not come about spontaneously, and which will continue subsequently, even when the child has been discharged from our Institute and has been integrated in a regular kindergarten or school. At its best, this process will result in a level of adjustment permitting him to function as a useful and contributing member of society, and this requires the development of language, attention, and diverse cognitive functions. However, society too must make an honest effort to accept the child who tries so hard to be admitted.

At least 60 per cent of the children at our Institute manage to attain the behavioural and academic standards set by the State system of education for average or below-average children. They are able to attend State schools and do not require specialised education for the severely handicapped. They avoid being institutionalised and do not require special equipment, even for writing or as a substitute for defective speech.

The Institute functions within the general education network of the country. It provides a formal education for school-age and preschool children, meeting the requirements set for all children in Hungary. Therefore a child can be transferred from the Institute to kindergarten or school only when the receiving school is convinced that he has attained these nationwide standards. When the Institute fails to provide convincing evidence, the school has the right to deny admission. Therefore we strive to maintain close contacts with governmental health, education and welfare services so as to make physicians, teachers, psychologists, social workers and physiotherapists aware of our ideas about the education of physically handicapped children.

The nature of Conductive Education

Our Institute is much closer to institutions offering education than to those providing therapy. CE is a system organised to maintain the continuity and coherence required by the educator. Within the system, it is the conductor who designs, organises and carries into effect the educational programme. She also serves as the contact-person for the supporting specialised services that will make their contributions *via* the conductor. By acting as an intermediary, the conductor prevents the fragmentation of the child and tends to lower the rigid boundaries among the professions.

The system fosters the conductor's autonomy. For any one child she can schedule the various sessions of the daily programme in such a way that the components each make significant contributions, while the unity of the whole is maintained. She can establish skills and plan for their application. She will ensure that a unity is formed between academic subjects and developing physical competencies.

Key elements in the organisation of the system of CE are: (i) the careful grouping, for the purposes of instruction, of the pupils on the basis of several criteria; (ii) the highly perfected team-work of the conductors and the conductors-in-training; and (iii) the nature of the interpersonal relations among the conductors themselves and the pupils in their care. Basic to these key elements is the fact that the Institute that delivers services also functions as the Conductor's College, the institution responsible for the professional training of all personnel ever to be employed in CE. This ensures a uniformity of outlook, philosophy and practical applications, which unfortunately too often is lacking in schools, clinics or hospitals elsewhere.

CE is an all-embracing system with its own register of those who one day may require care; its own diagnostic services, counselling services for parents, and client-centred services on the premises of the Institute; follow-up services for those transferred to kindergarten, school or a place of work; together with consultative services to the institutions that have received graduates from the Institute. This organisational network spans the whole of Hungary.

Conductors use teaching methods to reach the goals they set, and consequently the Institute comes under the Ministry of Education. The curriculum, timetable and methods of teaching are all shaped by the conductor to ensure that the child achieves, through learning activities, the intended eventual outcome. In essence, CE is no different in this respect from general education. Underlying this approach is the notion that for compensation or rehabilitation to take place, a creative process is needed in which the central nervous system will be permitted to restructure itself. Every person enrolled in CE, whether infant or adult, must develop his own method linking his executive and conative functions, *i.e.* linking what he does to what he wants to do. In order to reach this objective the programme cannot and does not depend primarily on practice and repetition.

Treatment

The word 'treatment' is actually a misnomer, since the Institute hopes to facilitate learning rather than to offer treatment. It is when a person learns to learn—and this applies to motor skills, balance, sensory and perceptual functions, emotional development, language and various cognitive functions—that we are reminded of the Oriental saying that if one gives a fish to a hungry man he will be saved from starvation today, but if one teaches him to fish, he and his family will prosper and be happy for life.

The programme must foster in the child a sense of personal responsibility and commitment. We do not deny the need to teach the elementary skills and competencies that normal children acquire without a great deal of instruction by trained personnel, but we feel that we should also reach for something much higher: learning to live through learning to learn. As a first step, we seek to establish contact and to stimulate the child to become an active participant in his process of education.

It is the conductor's responsibility to draw up the pupil's programme, carefully apportioning the various activities and their integration into the daily timetable, in line with the needs of the child and his future educational or vocational goals. All aspects of everyday living are included. There are opportunities for learning sensorimotor skills, self-care skills and general intellectual competencies, as well as those pre-academic skills required for success in state schools. In every teaching/ learning session, however, there are opportunities for the child to develop his own lifestyle, his own approach.

Special goals frequently serve as ends and at the same time as means to a more general goal. Locomotion, self-care and communication skills may be goals desirable in themselves, but once attained become means to a more comprehensive goal. Similarly, the possibility of leading an active life, having a healthy personal development, mutually beneficial family relationships and social esteem earned through achievement are goals of CE, but at the same time are important as positive reinforcers.

In CE the road towards the acquisition of an isolated skill runs *via* a training aimed at a more comprehensive goal, which then will include the targeted skill. For example, if the conductor tells a child to straighten out a bent arm or wrist, he cannot do it. If she tells him to hit a nail with a hammer, he will rapidly learn the movement the conductor wished to see established. It is also important that the conductor employs many tasks similar to the one of hammering the nail, for instance holding a stick and pretending it is a hammer, which is used to hit an imaginary nail, or other functionally related tasks.

The brain will institute and organise those activities that are relevant to the particular person. Feedback on the quality of performance is important, since it will enable the brain to restructure itself on the basis of this information, which means that the person is learning. Involving the child in learning activities that are relevant to his way of life will encourage the brain to restructure itself. At the same time, however, overt behaviour may be modified as well. It has frequently been noticed that when a tense person plans a relevant activity the process enables him to relax generally, whereas simple locomotion exercises, when they are felt to be irrelevant, may well produce increased tension.

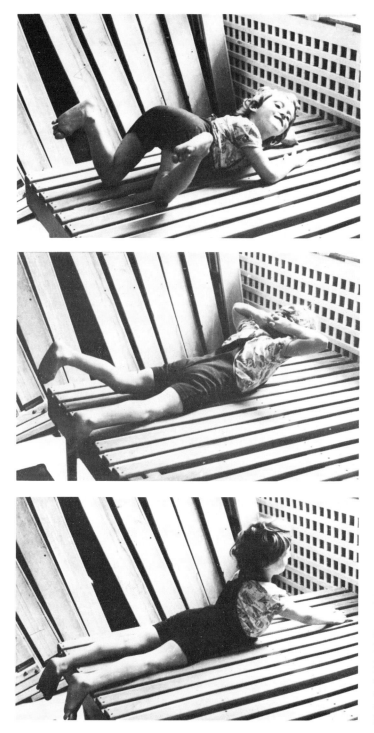

Fig. 1. A child on a plinth working in a lying task series. *Top:* beginning of task series, showing typical pathological posture. *Middle and bottom:* 30 minutes later, on completion of the task series. Child has been able to re-organise her posture on her own.

23

The conductor is expected to ensure that the several skills and competencies, while taught in a variety of ways, are properly integrated in the programme. Various teaching methods do not preclude each other and may be used simultaneously, as long as the idea of the whole is maintained. This is discussed under the next three sub-headings.

Movement for learning. Movement is regarded as one contributor to learning. The conductor at all times will stimulate active exploration of the world through movement. It is important that this active exploration should be rewarding to the child, because the child who has learned to explore successfully through purposeful activity will also develop a healthy and positive self-concept.

Underlying abilities. According to many authors (as reviewed by Ysseldyke and Salvia 1974) there are basic or underlying abilities which are prerequisites to success in academic subjects or their formal instruction. We would include attention, and the ability to translate intentions into intended overt behaviour. In this behaviour tensing and relaxing are subsumed, just as the pitch in music is governed by the tensing or relaxing of the strings. In a musical performance, however, the musician does not require conscious cortical control of the motor skills needed for each separate note. Some other underlying abilities are co-ordination and integration of functions, and sequential movement.

The concept of underlying abilities, as used here, means more than is commonly understood in Western countries. The abilities are not prerequisites in a temporal sense, but in a functional sense. They are subsumed under or embedded in the targeted skill. Conversely, whenever the whole or targeted skill is employed, the underlying abilities necessarily will be involved and therefore the use of the whole will contribute to the improvement and maintenance of the parts.

The approach followed is supported by views of human development which regard the whole as the framework within which the process of differentiation is constantly taking place. This is quite different from the block-building model, common in education, which sees the whole emerge from blocks being put one on top of the other.

To develop underlying abilities the training should make use of activities in which the underlying abilities are embedded, rather than attempt to develop these abilities separately. In our Institute it is felt that the cortex can deal with the underlying ability only when it is subsumed under the total skill, which will make it meaningful and relevant. Specific training, as advocated by Frostig or Kephart, for example, is not used in the Institute, since it is felt that perceptual and motor skills are already embedded in more complex or more complete skills which, because they are meaningful, offer much better opportunities for learning since a greater part of the cortex will be involved.

Task analysis. The training of underlying abilities does not preclude the task-analysis approach. This approach, commonly found in programmed learning, divides the tasks to be learned into a series of small steps which, taken in sequence, lead to the mastery of a complex routine. Developmental scales may be used to determine the order of the individual steps to be taken. Frequently the task-analysis model is considered to be the opposite of the underlying abilities model, but in our view they are not mutually exclusive because the underlying abilities, which are part of a whole function, interact with the whole to their mutual benefit. Within the framework of the whole, when the parts are permitted to vary, the common elements in the parts stress what is the same.

In task-analysis, the teaching sessions take the child from where he is to the aimed result *directly*, not by means of sub-skills deemed essential—whether the skill to be mastered is lying down, sitting, or standing. The skill is reviewed and further developed every day in an ascending spiral, which constantly brings the child's performance closer to the desired level. The practice of the whole skill then will also contribute to the acquisition of the parts, because the underlying skills are always involved in one form or another. Similarly, the tasks that make up the curriculum of the school form a longitudinal series, the sequence of which is given, but not the amount of time to be allotted to any one step. Steps are always linked, and the conductor will avoid any that are unrelated or meaningless. When the conductor, in order to ensure successful performance at the lowest level of the task-series, concludes that preliminary links are needed to prepare the child for the first step in the series, she may choose learning experiences which at first do not appear to be relevant. They may be similar to, analogous with, or even contrasting with the experiences of the first level. The clarifications or illustrations used to link steps will become less numerous as the series proceeds, and actual mastery of what must be learned will predominate more and more. Even if the form appears to be different, the function is essentially preserved.

Selection of groups
This is done by observing certain salient characteristics in the children and determining their relationship to the programme. A group comes into being through a consideration of several characteristics of the children. Selection for group-membership is a process of examining and re-examining children on diverse measures. The group must be large enough to permit individual differences and the formation of sub-groups around similarities. It must create a favourable climate for teacher-student and student-student interaction. It must ensure success. Working in a group is more than merely training group spirit and a sense of responsibility for others: it sets the stage for activities in which the members of the group learn to find ways to solve their problems. Each member of the group will go through the same series, but there will be variation in the time needed, the method employed and the level of performance attained; however, each will attain his maximum and his own way of solving problems the sub-tasks present.

To prevent one child from being singled out for unfavourable comment, the prevention or correction of incorrect behaviour is always directed towards the whole group, not to one child by name. But the child must be made to realise that the statement relates to him, if necessary with the help of a second conductor. However, children *are* singled out for praise. The conductor emphasizes what has

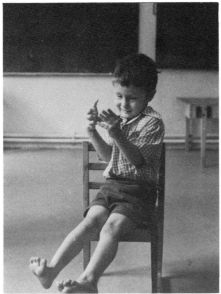

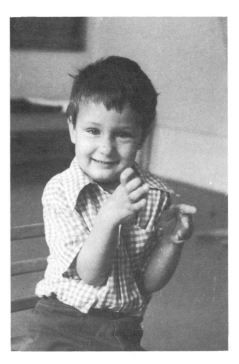

Fig. 2. *Above and right:* a child shows how he can *move* his fingers. *Below:* one year later, he has learned to *use* his hands.

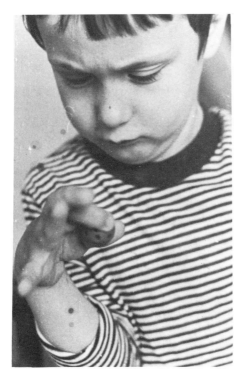

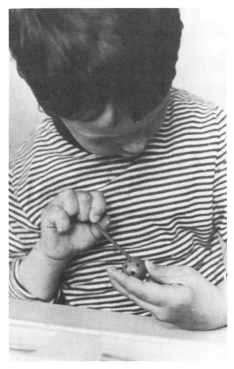

been accomplished so far, not where the child has failed. This positive approach enables the child to attempt to solve what is ahead of him confidently and independently.

The situation is different when a child has begun a movement but cannot go beyond the half-way point and is in danger of falling back to where he started. If failure is imminent, the conductor must help the child to succeed by offering a minimum of appropriate help, thus preventing a sense of failure and allowing him to give himself credit for the completion of the learning task.

The conductor does not present the pupils with the tasks to be learned, but accompanies the children in their progression through these steps which, as much as possible, are taken by the child independently. CE has nothing in common with, for example, practising musical scales or any other automatic motor skill: the conductor is able to monitor the unfolding of the programme and to combine, change or modify parts of it as she sees fit. She will also see to it that a proper balance is maintained between the introduction of new skills and the application of ones already established, and that they reinforce each other.

The integrative, spiralling effect is very important, and all previously acquired skills are included in each day's learning sessions. When a child has mastered a certain task, the skill needed for solving this problem will return as part of a more complex task, incorporated in a much wider context. This applies, for example, to the basic patterns of lying down, sitting, standing, prehension and speech, which will be used repeatedly, even during recess-periods between teaching sessions. Tasks are set by the conductor in such a way that the children use their skills at first consciously, then without being aware of doing so.

Through observation of the children in a large variety of settings, many of them practical life-situations, the conductor gathers information about the children's deficiencies or dysfunctions. This enables her to revise the programme of prerequisite skills and competencies by analysing the tasks and the ways of dissolving them into their component steps, which then are carefully graduated according to level of difficulty. Any situation in which the child happens to be can be used for observation and can serve as a point of departure for fruitful teaching.

Orthofunction
While it is important that the pupil works all through the day on the competencies that he will need, it is even more important that he finds the approach that is the most advantageous to him, *i.e.* his orthofunction. While engaged in solving the many tasks in the series, he discovers the methods most appropriate to him. The conductor will assist him in the discovery, but will not provide him with a solution. However, the conductor will try to prevent the establishment of inappropriate, self-defeating or improper approaches.

In order to be able to overcome the many barriers that our pupils no doubt will have to face in life, we must foster in the children a self-directed, spontaneous integration of correct approaches. To be challenging to the child and thus involve an important part of the cortex, the tasks should be quite difficult.

Orthofunction is quite difficult to define, but it includes: (i) the integration of what has been learned so far, as separate items; (ii) a person's best performance to date achieved without the use of a by-pass (an aid which replaces, rather than assists, the original function); and (iii) the avoidance of stereotyped, pathological behaviour and the adoption of healthy behaviour.

Pető regarded orthofunction as the opposite of dysfunction. While dysfunction is characterised by substandard or improper co-ordination or socially unacceptable behaviour, orthofunction is what is good and acceptable for a particular person. It is the function that his brain has constructed under the guidance of the conductor in order to cope with his situation. It should be judged on its qualities as a coping mechanism, not in terms of preconceived, socially determined criteria applicable to or derived from the performance of others.

The programme

In drawing up the programme, all dysfunctioning areas should be included and one should specify how much attention should be given to each. The timetable should state the time needed for everyday life skills and for teaching academic subjects—these two being parts of one whole. The programme indicates how and where differing goals may be pursued simultaneously. It is multidisciplinary, dealing simultaneously with different aspects of development. Thus language and movement might be combined to their mutual benefit, when movement supports the learning of language and the child's speech is used to control movement. For this to be possible, motor and speech development have to be planned as a unit. It is important to keep in mind the many-faceted nature of the learning, and the interrelatedness of the various tasks to be mastered. Even in planning one single lesson, we must ensure that opportunity is given to use the basic skills which have been learned, so that now they can be used automatically. Whatever is to be learned can be incorporated in different series of tasks and included in varying programmes.

Learning activities

The timetable should include not only what the curriculum requires to be taught, but particularly what contributes to maintaining a good mood and attitude and persistent attention. Therefore the daily programme includes short, alternating periods of different activities, which gradually can become longer. Such detailed planning does not preclude improvisation. The conductors can change the sequence, or prolong or shorten sessions, as the situation requires. For each specific subject, whether it be language, reading or writing, the series of tasks to be mastered is laid out in the spiral organisational pattern. The interaction among the learning processes directed to separate subject areas has a multiplying and integrating effect upon the child's total learning. The comprehensive nature of the programme fosters academic, social, aesthetic, ethical and emotional development. This highly organised curriculum, which draws from such a variety of disciplines, is perhaps an even greater contributor to the success of the Institute than its techniques or methodologies, however outstanding those may be.

28

The importance of flexibility
A flexible timetable is needed to extend the programme to include much more than the designated sessions. Time is a very important ingredient in the process of learning: it is needed for locomotion, communication and motor activities, to be practised throughout the day. Time must be made available for the acquisition of such self-care functions as locomotion and toilet-training in an unhurried fashion. In primary and secondary school, handicapped children frequently are not encouraged to go to the blackboard, but are kept in their wheelchairs, since it is thought that their slow movement takes too much time away from scheduled instruction. In such schools, academic subjects dominate the curriculum and little time is allowed for non-academic education, however vital it may be for some of the children. If a conductor decides there is not enough room in the therapeutic programme, she may incorporate these non-academic elements in the recreational programme, which is entirely controlled by the Institute. Visitors sometimes wonder whether our children have any leisure time at all, but the balanced development and high activity levels these children demonstrate shows that such an integrated programme does lead to a full life.

The conductor's autonomy and flexibility are much greater than those generally granted to teachers in ordinary schools. The conductor can incorporate any type of learning, academic or non-academic, recreational or emotional, and it is not necessary to assign special slots for them in the timetable. She is free to use any opportunity for contributing to the child's whole development.

Strategies and techniques
CE will help a child to find his own level of functioning, in line with his orthofunction. This means that he will establish a new pattern of skills and competencies which is best for him, although the pattern may be quite different from those of other or normal children.

In order to learn appropriate motor, sensorimotor and autonomic organisations, or to unlearn previously acquired inappropriate ones, the children in our Institute must go through a series of 'tasks' which will enable them to acquire substitute organisation. One strategy is for the conductor to help the child in areas that are not central to the learning task. For example, if the child has to reach for a chair with his right hand, the conductor may stabilise his legs, if necessary. The conductor may also help by constructing an alternative route which the child learns to follow. The child who cannot move his hand to his head can be shown an in-between position, in which his bent arm rests on his knee: he will stabilize his arm on his knee, move his head onto his hand, then bring head and arm, which remain connected, to an erect position. This type of help is allowed, because subsequently the child can incorporate it into his own repertoire.

Any support used in carrying out a movement should just be an aid. For instance when a child uses a chair for support, he should feel that his own legs carry more of his weight than the chair does, to ensure sufficient kinesthetic and visual feedback and so that he can experience the results of his own effort. In our pedagogy we include anything that will facilitate learning, as long as it is directed to

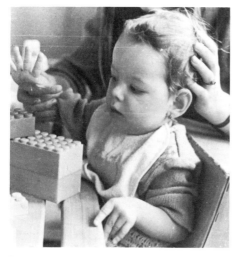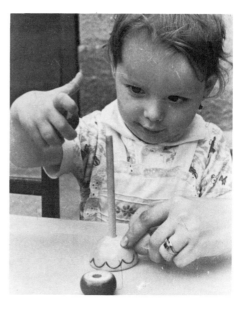

Fig. 3. Playing, learning grasp and release with manual assistance. *Left:* helping the child himself. *Right:* one year later, fixing the object only.

the formulated goals, is related to the child's previous learning, and fits the characteristics of the individual child. The conductor has at her disposal a wide variety of approaches, which at first sight appear to be 'techniques', but in CE are better described as 'experiences':

(1) to establish proper balance in a sitting or standing position;

(2) to control raising of arms or legs by using a base or 'anchor' to prevent unwanted movement;

(3) to stretch the arms in the desired direction and extend the range of movements;

(4) to enable the eyes to check or monitor movement;

(5) to make goals concrete instead of abstract;

(6) to improve or maintain posture;

(7) to allow the elbow or the back to be straightened.

The 'learning experiences' or approaches the conductor chooses to use serve also to stretch joints, to stabilise body-parts not essential to the process of learning, and to free or control movement in body-parts which are central to learning. Not only special equipment, but also certain parts of the body, can serve as props or pivots, provided the child learns to use them as such. Props or supports are considered as teaching-learning aids. Special equipment is a last resort and is allowable only if used temporarily, if it helps to teach skills not readily learned otherwise, and if used to prevent the formation of an incorrect body-image.

Gravity is one useful substitute for mechanical aids. In the standing position, gravity helps to maintain a limb in a stretched position. This process is called active fixation. Gravity also is used to maintain a limb in the extended position, or when a limb is allowed to swing freely without any active muscle involvement. The application of heat, or heat-producing ointments, may also be useful.

30

A dynamic aid is the resistance experienced when movement is directed against something. A synthetic aid is produced when several movements are combined, for instance as in lifting an arm, when the trunk can be rotated to facilitate abduction of the lower limb. A synthetic approach can also be used to teach posture, combining information obtained through all the senses with that received from the neck and labyrinth, to establish or maintain balance.

Effective learning is promoted by daily continuity of the programme, the specific sequence of tasks chosen from one or more of the task series, and by association of functions to be acquired: associating toilet-training, for instance, with certain colours, sounds or situations. It is worth repeating that when the child himself discovers the solution to his problem, the success of his endeavours will greatly assist his learning.

Rhythmic intention
What has been described so far as contributing to learning, forms a functional series linked with the intention of the person. When these contributors to learning are arranged in a series, subordinated to a formulated goal, 'rhythmic intention' comes about. Rhythmic intention is the person's mental preparation, *via* a symbolic representation, for overt behaviour. It professes that while initially the conductor states what is going to be the child's guiding principle, the latter will gradually take over the rôle of announcing what he will do and of carrying it out. When the conductor starts by saying, 'One, two, I hold it', she uses the word 'I', not 'you'. This helps to underline the fact that the child (repeating the 'I') is the principal actor in the scene.

The task, though chosen by the conductor, immediately becomes a shared commitment of both child and conductor, and in the course of time becomes the child's personal responsibility. In the learning-teaching session the conductor has to fade more and more into the background, the child increasingly occupying the centre of the stage. For this transfer to take place, the dysfunctional person must have such confidence in the conductor as to accept the goal-directed activity she has selected, and be willing to commit himself increasingly to the realisation of this goal. This requires that strong interest and lasting motivation are aroused in the child. It is part of the conductor's job to formulate the goal, to select the proper roads leading to its realisation, and to state these intended activities in words. The words must express what the child is to think, and therefore must represent or complement the child's thinking.

It has been found helpful to teach sequence and rhythm while the child says the directions. The intention, which is built on the words, is then harnessed to control the child's overt behaviour. In the case of aphasic patients, when speaking is difficult or impossible, control of overt behaviour is established by enlisting the help of another part of the body—arms or legs for example—which in turn will have a beneficial effect upon the person's ability to speak.

Every skill, including those involved in speaking, requires a well-developed sequencing of rhythmic actions. The ability to analyse and to carry out this sequence is gradually controlled by the person himself. This is because intention, initially conscious, will eventually lead to an unconscious control of the sequencing process. In turn the spoken word may itself encourage other sequencing processes.

Integration into society

Integrating the physically handicapped with the rest of society is one of the main aims of CE. At the Institute we do not consider our task finished when the child has acquired certain motor patterns and learned to use them. We also deem it necessary to make careful preparations for the child's transition from the Institute to a kindergarten or state school. These preparations include modifying the child's daily routine to fit in with the school; and we gradually increase the hourly load so that the child will be able to meet the demands of the school's timetable.

An elaborate system of follow-up services ensures that once the child has left the Institute he is not allowed to stagnate or slide back. When a child has been admitted to a school or kindergarten, a conductor will visit the school to observe him in the new environment, at first once every three months but gradually less frequently if all goes well. She will spend time in the child's classroom, check up on his adjustment, watch out for any regression, and consult with the principal and the teachers. If necessary, the itinerant conductor can arrange for the child to return to the Institute at the end of the school year for a short refresher course.

Apart from this follow-up service, which reaches deep into the school system, the Institute also maintains liaisons with the consultative and supportive services of the school system, with the medical services attached to the schools, and with the network of social workers.

Summary

The Institute should be regarded primarily as an educational agency which uses a multitude of approaches and techniques to realise educational goals. It seeks to integrate the physically handicapped as active participators in our society. It uses a programme that is undoubtedly multidisciplinary in character, but which manages to avoid the damaging fragmentation of the child, because it integrates all contributions through the conductor, who serves as the mediator between the supportive services and the child.

We gratefully acknowledge the help received from the International Cerebral Palsy Society. Special thanks are due to Mr J. Loring, who has supported conductive Education for many years. We also wish to express our gratitude to Mrs Esther Cotton, for her untiring efforts.
Professor Tillemans's participation was facilitated by support from the SSHRC of Canada and the Hungarian Academy of Sciences.

REFERENCE

Ysseldyke, J. E., Salvia, J. (1974) 'Diagnostic-prescriptive teaching: two models.' *Exceptional Children,* **41**, 181–185.

FURTHER READING

Ákos, K. (1975) *Az Idők Örvényében.* Budapest: Gondolat.

Bernklau, K. O. (1965) *Unfug der Krankheit. Triumpf der Heilkunst.* Hanau Main: Karl Schustek.
Bosch, J. de la Pena (1972) *Problemas de la Parálisis Cerébral y su Tratemiento.* Madrid: Real Academia National de Medicine.
Bowley, A. H., Gardner, L. (1980) *The Handicapped Child. 4th Edn.* Edinburgh: Churchill Livingstone.
Biró, K. (1971) 'Nevelők nevelése a konduktorképzés során.' *Felsőoktatási Szemle,* **20,** 487–490.
Carrington, M. E. (1974) 'An appraisal of assessment and treatment techniques for the care of handicapped children in Europe.' *Physiotherapy,* **60,** 315–322.
Clarke, J., Evans, E. (1973) 'Rhythmical intention as a method of treatment for the cerebral palsied patient.' *Australian Journal of Physiotherapy,* **19,** 57–64.
Cotton, E. (1965) 'The Institute for Movement Therapy and School for "Conductors", Budapest, Hungary.' *Developmental Medicine and Child Neurology,* **17,** 437–446.
—— (1969) 'Conductive Education with special reference to severe athetoids in a non-residential centre.' *Journal of Mental Subnormality,* **14**(1), 50–56.
—— (1970) 'Integration of treatment and education in cerebral palsy.' *Physiotherapy,* **56,** 143–147.
—— (1974) 'Improvement in motor function with the use of Conductive Education.' *Developmental Medicine and Child Neurology,* **16,** 637–643.
—— (1975, 1977) *Conductive Education and Cerebral Palsy.* London: The Spastics Society.
—— (1975) 'Disturbances of higher nervous activity in hemiplegia.' *Physiotherapy,* **61,** 341.
—— (1976) *Pető Unit 1.* London: The Spastics Society.
—— (1976) *The Basic Motor Pattern. 2nd Edn.* London: The Spastics Society.
—— (1981) *The Hand as a Guide to Learning.* London: The Spastics Society.
—— Parnwell, M. (1967) 'From Hungary: the Pető method.' *Special Education,* **56,** 7.
Cruickshank, W. M. (Ed.) (1976) *Cerebral Palsy. A Developmental Disability. 3rd Edn.* Syracuse, N.Y.: Syracuse University Press.
Diehl, H. J. (1982) 'Rehabilitation im Ausland.' *Die Rehabilitation,* **21,** 76–77.
Eckhardt, H. (1964) 'Die behandlung cerebralgelähmter kinder in der bewegungsversehrten erziehungsanstalt und konduktorseminar Budapest under der leitung von Prof. Pető.' *Beiträge zur Orthopädie und Traumatologie,* **11,** 419–424.
—— (1964) 'Orthopaedische probleme beim spastisch gelähmten kind.' *Beiträge zur Orthopädie und Traumatologie,* **11,** 825–830.
Feldkamp, M., Danielcik, I. (1976) *Krankengymnastisch Behandlung der Cerebralen Bewegungsstörung (2nd Edn.).* München: R. Pflaum.
Gardner, L. (1968) *Suggestion on the Development of the Pető Method.* London: The Spastics Society.
—— (1968) *Report of Sub-Group on Pető Method of Conductive Education.* London: The Spastics Society.
Gegesi, K. P. (1966) 'A gyermeki pszyche fejlődése és a környezeti hatás néhány kérdése.' *Gyermekgyógyászat,* **7,** 33–51.
Gordon, N. (1976) *Pediatric Neurology for the Clinician. Clinics in Developmental Medicine Nos. 59/60.* London: S.I.M.P. with Heinemann; Philadelphia: Lippincott.
Halász, Z. (1965) 'Home-thoughts from across the Channel.' *New Hungarian Quarterly,* 110–113.
Hári, M. (1955) 'A fájdalom és a mozgásos kezelés.' Pavlov Ideg Elme Szakcsoport Nagygyülése, 1953. (Előadás) Ideggyógyászati Szemle 1955, évi melléklete, p. 230.
—— (1955) 'A spasztikus paraplégiák kezeléséről.' Pavlov Ideg Elme Szakcsoport Nagygyülése, 1953. (Előadás) Ideggyógyászati Szemle 1955, évi melléklete, p. 312.
—— (Ed.) (1962) *Bevezető a Konduktiv Mozgáspedagógiába Pető András előadásai alapján.* Budapest: Gyógypedagógiai Tanárképző Főiskola.
—— Székely, F. (1968) 'Konduktiv pedagógia.' *Köznevelés,* **24,** 493–494.
—— (1970) 'A mozgássérültek konduktiv pedagógiája.' *Magyar Tudomány,* **15,** 30–34.
—— Ákos, K. (1971) *Konduktiv Pedagógia 1.* Budapest: Tankönyvkiadó.
—— (1973) *A Dysfunkciós Gyermek és az Integráció.* Budapest: A Magyar Rehabilitációs Tarsaság Nagygyülése, X.12. 226.
—— (1973) 'Hozzászólas dr. Benczur Miklósné—László Emma "A mozgássérültek iskolai rehabilitálása" cimü cikkéhez.' *Gyógypedagógia,* **18,** 56–57.
—— (1974) 'Az elmélet és gyakorlat egysége a konduktorképzésben.' *Felsőoktatási Szemle,* **23,** 176–178.
—— (1976) 'A mozgássérültek testi nevelésének feladatai.' *In:* Nádori, L. (Ed.) *A sport és testnevelés időszerü kérdései,* **14,** 123–137.
—— (1977) 'A mozgássérültek helyzete a Szovjetunióban.' *Gyógypedagógia,* **22,** 91–94.

—— (1977) 'A magyarországi mozgássérültek konduktiv nevelőhálózata. Une analyse critique de la situation des handicapés moteurs en Hongrie.' Paris: *Les Nouvelles de l'UNESCO.*

—— (Ed.) (1977) *Feladatok és Módszerek Gyüjteménye 1.* Budapest: Mozgássérültek Nevelőképző és Nevelőintézete.

—— (Ed.) (1977) *Feladatok és Módszerek Gyüjteménye 2–3. Budapest: Mozgássérültek Nevelőképző és Nevelőintézete.*

—— (1977) 'Módszereiuk és eredményeink a mozgássérültek rehabilitációjában.' *Magyar Pediáter,* Supplementum 11. 70–75.

—— (1978) *Tünettan (Jegyzet).* Budapest: Mozgássérültek Nevelőképző és Nevelőintézete.

—— (Ed.) (1979) *Feladatok és Módszerek Gyüjteménye 4.* Budapest: Mozgássérültek Nevelőképző és Nevelőintézete.

—— (Ed.) (1979) *Feladatok és Módszerek Gyüjteménye 5.* Budapest: Mozgássérültek Nevelőképző és Nevelőintézete.

—— (Ed.) (1979) *Feladatok és Módszerek Gyüjteménye 6.* Budapest: Mozgássérültek Nevelőképző és Nevelőintézete.

—— (Ed.) (1980) *Feladatok és Módszerek Gyüjteménye 7.* Budapest: Mozgássérültek Nevelőképző és Nevelőintézete.

—— (1980) 'L'Éducation Conductive.' *Motricité Cérébrale,* **1,** 115–123.

—— (1980) 'Mit ismer meg a hallgató képzése folyamán?' *Konduktiv pedagógia 2/1.* Budapest: Mozgássérültek Nevelőképző és Nevelőintézete.

—— (1980) 'Mi szükséges a program felépitéséshez?' *Konduktive pedagógia 2/2.* Budapest: Mozgássérültek Nevelőképző és Nevelőintézete.

—— (1980) 'Lábfejmozgások, térdmozgások, csipőmozgások.' *Konduktiv pedagógia 2/3.* Budapest: Mozgássérültek Nevelőképző Nevelőképző és Nevelőintézete.

—— (Ed.) (1981) *Feladatok és Módszerek Gyüjteménye 8/1.* Budapest: Mozgássérültek Nevelőképző és Nevelőintézete.

—— (Ed.) (1981) *Feladatok és Módszerek Gyüjteménye 8/2.* Budapest: Mozgássérültek Nevelőképző és Nevelőintézete.

—— (1981) 'Az orthofunkció kialakitása.' *Konduktiv pedagógia 2/4.* Budapest: Mozgássérültek Nevelőképző és Nevelőintézete.

—— (1982) 'A konduktiv pedagógia lehetőségei a mozgássérültek rehabilitációjában' 21. Bács-Kiskun megyei Orvos- Gyógyszerész Napok 1981. Október 15–16. Kalocsa. Kecskemét: Bács-Kiskun megyei Orvosok—Gyógyszerészek Evkönyve, 1982. p. 21–27.

—— (1982) 'A konduktiv pedagógia rendszere és szerepe a központi idegrendszeri sérültek társadalmi beilleszkedésében.' *Gyermekgyógyászat,* **33,** 497–510.

—— (1982) 'Metod konduktivnoj pedagogiki i ego Rol' v Szocial'noj adaptacii bolnüh detszkim cerebralnüm paralicsom.' *Zhurnal Nevropatologii i Pszihiatrii,* **82,** 67–70.

Haskell, S., Barrett, E., Taylor, H. (1977) *The Education of Motor and Neurologically Handicapped Children.* London: Croom Helm.

Horváthné, B. A. (1982) 'Ki a konduktor?' *Megyei Pedagógiai Hiradó,* **12,** 40–41.

House, J. (1968) 'Breakthrough in Budapest. An interview with Professor James House about a method of helping severely disabled children.' *Ideas of Today,* **16,** 110–114.

—— (1971) *Evaluating an Integrated Approach to the Management of Cerebral Palsy.* Wisconsin: Wisconsin State University.

Holt, K. S. (1975) 'A single nurse-teacher-therapist?' *Child, Care, Health and Development,* **1,** 45–50.

Institute for Conductive Education of the Motor Disabled Conductor's College (1975) 'Scientific Studies on Conductive Pedagogy.' Budapest.

Jernquist, L. (1978) 'My head is in the middle.' *ICPS Bulletin* (January and Summer).

Kállay, Gy. (1981) Központi idegrendszeri sérült csecsemők fejlesztésének lehetőségei a Mozgássérültek Nevelőképző és Nevelőintézetében. Magyar Gyermekorvosok Társasága Délmagyarországi Decentruma tudományos Ülése, Makó, május 15. /Előadás./

Keresztes, J. (1977) 'Mozgássérültek szocializációja.' *Magyar Pediáter,* Supplementum 11, 77.

Klein, O. (1968) 'Zur vorbereitung zerebralgelähmter kinder auf den schulbesuch.' *Die Sonderschule, 1. Beiheft,* 16–52.

—— (1962) 'Zur bewegungspädagogischen behandlung cerebral gelähmter kinder im Institut Bewegungspädagogik, Budapest.' *Beiträge zur Orthopädie und Traumatologie,* **9,** 315–332.

Köng, E. (1974) *Cerebrale Bewegungsstörungen beim Kind.* Basel: Karger.

Kulakowski, S. (1982) *Traitement Neurologique Integré de l'Enfant Porteur d'une Atteinte Cérébrale.* Berck Plage.

34

Lehnhard, R. (1965) 'Lebenshilfe für Bewegungsversehrte.' *Deutsches Arzteblatt—Arztliche Mitteilungen*, **63**, 1–5.
—— (1966) 'Ein Modell aus Ungarn: Hilfe für Bewegungsversehrte.' *Das Behinderte Kind*, **2**, 115–117.
—— (1967) 'Rhytmisches Intendieren als Kern der Bewegungspädogogik.' *Medical Tribune*, **44**, 10–11.
Loring, J. (1971) 'A visit to the Pető Institute for Spastic Children in Budapest.' *New Hungarian Quarterly*, **12**, 140–143.
—— (1978) 'Integrated therapy education and child care.' *In:* Apley, J. (Ed.) *Care of the Handicapped Child. Clinics in Developmental Medicine No. 67.* London: S.I.M.P. with Heinemann; Philadelphia: Lippincott.
Moor, J. M. H. de (1977) *De Geintegreerde Behandeling van Gehandicapte Kinderen: Problemen en Mogelÿkheden.* Noordhoff Groningen: Wolters.
Mosolygó, D. (1974) 'A rehabilitáció helyzete és feladatai különös tekintettel az orvosi rehabilitációra.' *Népegészégügy*, **55**, 65–71.
Mozgásterápiai Intézet és Tanszék Munkaközössége, (1955) *Hemiplegia Gyakorlatok.* Budapest: Gyógypedagógiai Tanárképző Főiskola.
Mozgásterápiai Tanszék Munkaközössége, (1955) *Mozgásterápiai Irodalom gyüjtemény.* Budapest: Gyógypedagógiai Tanárképző Főiskola Mozgásterápiai Tanszéke.
—— (1956) *Utmutató.* Budapest: Gyógypedagógiai Tanárképző Főiskola.
Mozgásterápiai Intézet és Tanszék Közössége, (1957, 1959) *Mozgásterápiai Tájékoztató.* Budapest: Gyógypedagógiai Tanárképző Főiskola.
Mozgássérültek Nevelőképző és Nevelőintézete, (1971) *Tudományos Közlemények.* Budapest: MSI.
—— (1973) *Tudományos Közlemények.* Budapest: MSI.
Müller, L. (1972) 'Pető-Behandling af C.P.-born is Budapest.' *Tidskrift for Fysioterapeuter*, **54**, 353–358.
Oskamp, U. (1982) 'Therapie-not oder not-therapie.' *Zeitschrift für Heilpädagogik*, **33**, 590–592.
Pálfalvi, L. (1970) 'Perinatális cerebrális károsodások után hyperkinézisben szenvedők audiológiai vizsgálata és gondozása.' *Orvosi Hetilap*, **111**, 2948–2952.
Patzer, H. (1966) 'Organisation der erfassung und betreuung zerebralgelähmter kinder in ungarn.' *Mitteilungen Über Praxis und Probleme der Rehabilitation*, **2**, 4–13.
Pető, A. (1955) 'Konduktiv mozgásterápia mint gyógypedagógia.' *Gyógypedagógia*, **1**, 15–21.
Püschel, W. (1965) 'Lebenshilfe für bewegungsversehrte. Ungarn gibt ein modell für lösung.' *Naturheilpraxis, Heft* **10**.
Püski, É. (1977) 'Mozgássérült csecsemők konduktiv nevelése.' *Magyar Pediáter*, (Supplementum 11), 75–76.
Scrutton, D., Gilbertson, M. (1975) *Physiotherapy in Paediatric Practice.* London: Butterworths.
Siebbrandt, K. (1967) 'Hilfen für spastisch gelähmte kinder unter hinweis auf cerebralgelähmter kinder im Institut für Bewegungspädagogik in Budapest.' *Bildungsarbeit an Behinderten*, **5**.
Squire, C. (1982) 'New ideas on the case and treatment of strokes.' *British Journal of Occupational Therapy*, **45**, 266–267.
Szemenova, K., Masztjukova, E. (1974) 'O konduktivnom voszpitanii detej sz cerebralnümi paralicsami v vengerszkoj narodnoj reszpublike.' *Defektologija*, **2**, 93–95.
Ungvári, E., Schmidt, H. L. (1967) 'Bericht über das Institut für Bewegungstherapie in Budapest.' *Krankengymnastik*, **19**, 323–325.
Varty, E. (1970) 'Conductive Education.' *Physiotherapy*, **56**, 414–415.
—— (1972) 'A child's world—of specialists?' *Special Education*, **March,** 6–9.
—— (1973) 'What about the integrated child?' *Special Education*, **62**, 24–26.
Vizkelety, T. (1977) 'Orthopaediai mütétek szerepe a spastikus betegek kezelésében.' *Magyar Traumatológia*, **20**, 195–210.
—— (1980) 'Die tátigkeit des orthopäden im rahmen der Behandlungsmethode Pető.' *Orthopädische Praxis*, **16**, 270–272.
Woods, G. (Ed.) (1975) *The Handicapped Child.* Oxford: Blackwell.

3

HOME-BASED EARLY INTERVENTION: A DESCRIPTION OF THE PORTAGE PROJECT MODEL

George Jesien

Introduction

The Portage* Project was among the first to explore, study, and involve parents directly in the education and treatment of their young children with handicaps. The Project began in 1969, with funding from the Bureau for the Education of the Handicapped (now called Special Education Programs) of the US Office of Education under the Handicapped Children's Early Education Assistance Act. The purpose of this new legislation was to test and establish innovative early education programs for handicapped children, which might lead to comprehensive models that could be replicated by others. Selected programs were assured three years of funding for program development, implementation, and evaluation. After this period a program was expected to obtain local funding to continue services.

The project began with 48 children, aged up to three years old, with a variety of handicapping conditions—mental retardation, language delays, cerebral palsy, learning disabilities, physical handicaps, and behavioral problems. The model that evolved has the following characteristics (Shearer and Shearer 1976):

(1) The educational program takes place in each child's home and is implemented by a home teacher who visits each family weekly.

(2) Assessment procedures list the child's competencies, as a basis for preparing an individualized curriculum.

(3) Teaching methods are based on principles of applied behavior analysis.

(4) The curriculum is planned with the expectation that the child will achieve the prescribed goals weekly.

(5) Parents or the principal caregivers work with the child during the week, providing daily instruction.

(6) The teachers meet weekly, to discuss problems and modify the curriculum.

Evaluation studies of the initial model showed that children made significant gains in the acquisition of physical, cognitive, language, social, and self-help skills. Pre- and post-program comparisons on a variety of assessment instruments (Cattell Infant Intelligence Scale, Stanford-Binet Intelligence Scale, and the Alpern-Boll Developmental Profile) showed consistently greater gains for children receiving project services than could be expected based on previous developmental progress (Shearer and Shearer 1972). Furthermore, data comparing the performance of children receiving home visitation with those attending local classroom programs

*Portage is a town in Wisconsin, USA.

36

for culturally and economically disadvantaged preschoolers, showed a significant difference in favor of project children in terms of their mental age and IQ scores (Cattell Infant Intelligence Scale, Stanford-Binet Intelligence Scale, and Gessell Developmental Schedule), as well as in their language, academic, and socialization skills as measured by the Alpern-Boll Developmental Profile (Peniston 1972). The positive evaluation results and the high degree of parental satisfaction led to the local school districts funding the program when Federal funding for direct services terminated in 1972.

Replication evaluation results also indicated that the Portage Project might have promise as a model for early intervention in other rural areas in the US. In 1972, the Project received funds to test this possibility as an Outreach Project. The purpose of Outreach activities was to offer assistance to agencies interested in replicating the Portage Project and to evaluate the effectiveness of the replication process. Replication sites were chosen based on a variety of administrative structures and staffing patterns and funding sources including public schools, state and private institutions, hospitals, and Head Start* programs. The children included a wide variety of handicapping conditions and degrees of delay, ranging from profound to at risk of delay. In an attempt to test the proposed model further, both rural and urban sites were selected. Results showed that children in replication sites were making very similar gains to those at the original program (Portage Project 1975). The severity of handicapping condition and type of staff or administrative structure did not appear to mediate the magnitude of the effects. Professional teachers and trained paraprofessionals obtained similarly significant gains with their children (Schortinghuis and Frohman 1974). The critical factors appeared to be the regularly scheduled weekly home visits, the co-operation of parents with the home teacher, and a data-based decision-making process.

The Portage Home Intervention Model has been replicated extensively over the last 12 years, and there are now over 140 sites in the United States and Canada. However, over the last five years one of the major unforeseen activities of the Portage Project has been its involvement with early intervention programs in other countries. Interest in Portage procedures and materials has led to numerous adaptations for serving developmentally delayed or socio-economically disadvantaged children. Home visitors have ranged from nurses and other health workers to professional and paraprofessional preschool teachers. In a number of developing countries the Portage Model has been able to provide communities with a cadre of trained early interventionists (Thorburn 1981, Jesien 1983). As the result of a major effort to adapt the Portage Model to Latin American needs (Jesien *et al.* 1979) numerous programs in South America use the Spanish version of the *Portage Guide to Early Education* as a resource.

In Great Britain, two replication efforts in Winchester (Smith *et al.* 1977) and in Cardiff, Wales (Revill and Blunden 1979) have led to a growing interest in the Model and its materials (Cameron 1982). In 1983 the Third Portage Annual Conference was held in London and a National Portage Association was proposed

*Early intervention.

to support programs and professionals using the Portage scheme. Such an organization could prove to be valuable for testing adaptations and modifications of the Model in a variety of settings.

Rationale

The same basic assumptions have guided the Portage Project's efforts over the last 14 years:

(1) Intervention should begin as early as possible, to have the maximum effect on the child.

(2) Parents are the most powerful educators of their children. Regardless of their education, economic status, or intellectual capacity, they are the architects of their children's environment.

(3) The home is a natural and effective environment for working with the child and his/her family.

(4) An individualized developmentally-sequenced approach is the most effective for guiding pedagogical strategies and the development of curricular activities. Each child has a unique profile of strengths and weaknesses which need to be addressed.

(5) Finally, the focus of intervention should be neither the child nor the caregiver alone, but rather the interaction between child and parent. It is in this mutually reciprocal interaction that development is enhanced and guided.

Since 1969, thousands of handicapped children and their families have been served by the Portage Model in Wisconsin and other sites across the United States. These multi-agency experiences have pointed out a number of advantages inherent in the model (Shearer 1984):

(1) Behaviors selected for learning, as well as the teaching method, are likely to be highly functional since teaching and learning are occurring in the environment where behaviors will naturally be used and rewarded.

(2) The professional time spent with the parent provides a double return, in that the parent as well as the child learns the teaching skills. These skills will be practised on a long-term basis.

(3) The home teacher works on a one-to-one basis with parents and child, resulting in the individualization of instructional goals and teaching strategies for both. A wide variety and degree of handicapping conditions can, therefore, be given specific attention.

(4) Differences in familial lifestyles and cultural values can be accommodated by the program. Such modifications in the goals selected or in the teaching methods increase the practicality of behaviors learned.

(5) When parents directly participate in the intervention program, the child's learning rate is accelerated (Fredericks *et al.* 1976) and can have beneficial effects on siblings (Klaus and Gray 1968).

(6) Some of the emotional distress associated with having a child with a handicap can be alleviated. Regular visits by a teacher dedicated to the particular needs of child and family can provide the necessary support to parents as the family readjusts to their new situation.

Model description

The Portage Model has been adapted to meet the needs of particular child populations and administrative structures.

Screening and identification

The first component in the Portage Model is the identification and screening of children who may be eligible to receive the service. Each agency establishes its eligibility criteria depending upon its service population, governmental regulations, and the number of families that can be served. Eligibility criteria are typically stated in terms of the presence of a specific syndrome, documented developmental delay or IQ scores.

Health and educational agencies, health and social welfare practitioners and parents themselves are the most common sources of referral. The project's efforts have concentrated on informing the professional community of the availability of services and disseminating information on the need and importance of early intervention to the community at large. Eligible children have been located with the help of leaflets and local radio messages. Once a child is identified, the home teacher makes an appointment to visit the home. At the initial visit the home teacher explains the program, obtains permission to evaluate the child, and begins the assessment process. Some initial evaluation data may have already been collected if the child is referred from a health clinic or other agency.

Assessment

The assessment process aims to discover the unique strengths and weaknesses of a child, and so to improve that child's intervention program. The home teacher begins the process by administering formal standardized instruments such as the Developmental Profile II (Alpern *et al.* 1980), Peabody Picture Vocabulary, McCarthy Scales of Children's Abilities (1972) and any others that may be appropriate depending on the functioning level of the child and the handicapping condition. Other members of the multidisciplinary team may conduct in-depth evaluations in the deficit areas.

If possible, evaluation of the child takes place in the home with the parents present. This may be difficult to do in some instances, but a much more reliable data sample is obtained in surroundings familiar to the child. Also the parents, who know the child best, are involved in the evaluation process from the beginning. This establishes a pattern of participation which will be essential to the intervention process. Experience has shown that when parents are involved in the evaluation phase, they are more ready and capable of participating in the intervention phases. The teacher also observes any environmental and teaching factors which will be most conducive to learning. The teacher gives the child an opportunity to react to numerous materials during various activities to ascertain the child's learning style, frustration tolerance, response to reinforcement and correction procedures and other situation-specific factors that will assist in planning future instructional activities.

Age Level	Card	Behavior	Entry Behavior	Date Achieved	Comments
0-1	1	Removes cloth from face. that obscures vision		/ /	
	2	Looks for object that has been removed from direct line of vision		/ /	
	3	Removes object from open container by reaching into container		/ /	
	4	Places object in container in imitation		/ /	
	5	Places object in container on verbal command		/ /	
	6	Shakes a sound making toy on a string		/ /	
	7	Puts 3 objects into a container, empties container		/ /	
	8	Transfers object from one hand to the other to pick up another object		/ /	
	9	Drops and picks up toy		/ /	
	10	Finds object hidden under container		/ /	
	11	Pushes 3 blocks train style		/ /	
	12	Removes circle from form board		/ /	
	13	Places round peg in pegboard on request		/ /	
	14	Performs simple gestures on request		/ /	
1-2	15	Individually takes out 6 objects from container		/ /	
	16	Points to one body part		/ /	
	17	Stacks 3 blocks on request		/ /	
	18	Matches like objects		/ /	
	19	Scribbles		/ /	
	20	Points to self when asked "Where's (name)?"		/ /	
	21	Places 5 round pegs in pegboard on request		/ /	
	22	Matches objects with picture of same object		/ /	
	23	Points to named picture		/ /	
	24	Turns pages of book 2-3 at a time to find named picture		/ /	
2-3	25	Finds specific book on request		/ /	
	26	Completes 3 piece formboard		/ /	
	27	Names 4 common pictures		/ /	

PortageGuide

Fig. 1. Part of the Developmental Sequence Checklist for assessing cognitive skills (© Cooperative Educational Service Agency 12).

Individual educational plan

Results of the initial evaluation and any pertinent historical information are brought together in the Individual Educational Plan (IEP) Meeting. By US law, each special-needs child must have an IEP delineating the child's immediate and long-term intervention goals. The plan also contains details of any ancillary services that the child will need, such as occupational or physical therapy, and the respective responsibilities of the professional involved in providing services to the child and family. Parents participate in the meeting and must agree to the plan before it can be put into effect. Since parents have already participated in the evaluation process, they can be more realistically expected to participate in the planning process. The IEP serves as a blueprint for guiding intervention and the selection of curricular activities.

Curriculum planning

To assist in the planning of weekly goals, based on the child's present functioning level, the Portage staff developed the *Portage Guide to Early Education* (Bluma *et al.* 1976). The guide consists of three parts:

(1) The manual describes the developmental areas covered in the guide: infant stimulation, cognition, language, motor, socialization, and self-help. It also contains directions for using the guide and for planning and implementing instructional activities.

(2) The Developmental Sequence Checklist contains 580 developmentally sequenced skills in the six areas of development from zero to six years (Fig. 1).

(3) The Curriculum Card File lists four to seven possible ways of teaching each of the 580 skills (Fig. 2).

The purpose of the *Portage Guide to Early Education* is to assist the teacher and parents to identify those behaviors and skills which the child has already acquired and those which the child is prepared to learn next—called emerging behaviors. This is accomplished by administering the Checklist in each of the curriculum areas before the intervention program begins. The child's performance, coupled with information supplied by the parent or principal caregiver, provides the teacher with information on which behaviors to select for teaching. In addition, parental requests, results from the initial evaluation, and the child's short-term and long-term goals from the IEP are taken into account when planning the child's instructional program.

Because children will not necessarily follow the sequence of skills in the Checklist, it should not be applied rigidly. Fully 50 per cent of the behaviors selected for children are not found in the Checklist but may be skills leading to the accquisition of behaviors on the Checklist. The severity of a child's delay or the type of handicapping condition may require that goals be broken down into very small steps which are worked on weekly. A child who has limited use or control of parts of his/her body may have to have Checklist goals modified or even eliminated. The Guide will provide a fairly accurate profile of the child's present skills repertoire and provide a number of alternatives for the next steps in teaching.

The Card File provides alternative activities and suggested materials for

AGE 1-2

TITLE: Matches objects with picture of some object

WHAT TO DO:

1. Cut and mount toy pictures from catalog that look similar to child's own toys. Give child a doll, ask child to find the picture of the doll. Repeat for any familiar object.
2. Hold up picture of object and say "here's a _____ . You find the other _____."
   Help him if necessary by showing him which object goes with the pictures. Continue until child can match the pictures and objects unassisted.
3. Cut out pictures of food or food cans and boxes from magazines. Let child try to match them to the actual product in your refrigerator or on the shelves.
4. If the child is having difficulty, take photographs of his own toys and real household objects with which he is familiar. Have him match the real object with a real picture of it. Later let him match objects to line drawings.

PortageGuide

© 1976 Cooperative Educational Service Agency 12

AGE 2-3

TITLE: Takes off simple clothing that has been unfastened

WHAT TO DO:

1. Make it a nightly responsibility of the child to remove dress or pants. Continue to encourage and let the child practice. Compliment child on being a big boy (or girl).
2. Give child a sticker to put on chart each time he takes off clothing without help.
3. Practice undressing dolls.
4. Don't expect the child to undress himself completely at first. Start with one or two items. When he masters these add another item.
5. Regardless of what clothing item you choose to begin teaching give the child physical aid with verbal directions. Gradually withdraw the physical and verbal help as the child gains in skill.

PortageGuide

© 1976 Cooperative Educational Service Agency 12

Fig. 2. Extracts from the Curriculum Card File.

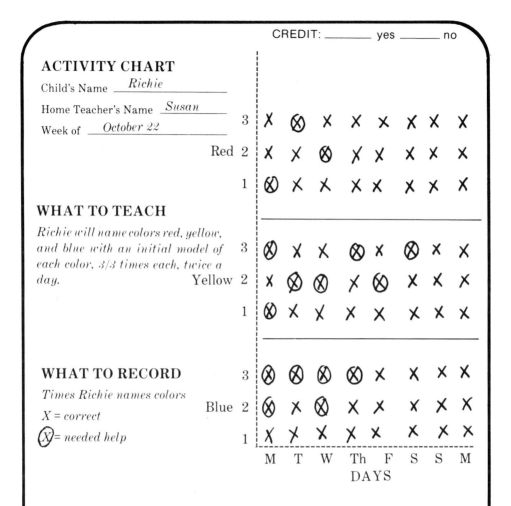

ACTIVITY CHART

Child's Name _____Richie_____

Home Teacher's Name _____Susan_____

Week of _____October 22_____

WHAT TO TEACH

Richie will name colors red, yellow, and blue with an initial model of each color, 3/3 times each, twice a day.

WHAT TO RECORD

Times Richie names colors

X = correct

Ⓧ = needed help

DIRECTIONS

Use colored chips. Place a chip of each color on the table. Name the color as you do this. Have Richie repeat each color after you. Then hold up a chip and ask "What color is this?" When Richie answers correctly, praise and give him a small circle of the same color. Mark the response with X. If he is incorrect, ask him "Is this red, yellow or blue?" Mark this response with Ⓧ . Mix up the order as you ask for the colors. Do this activity once in the morning and once in the afternoon, but only record the answers from the morning.

Fig. 3. Completed activity chart.

teaching each of the skills in the Checklist. Each of the suggestions has been found to be useful in teaching special-needs children. These too may need to be modified depending upon the instructional context and the particular needs of the child.

The entire Portage system can be used in conjunction with other curricular materials and treatment procedures. Many programs have used the curriculum guide as the mainstay of their developmental program while others choose to use it as an additional resource for their teachers. The latter approach is especially appropriate for programs that deal with a particular handicap; the curriculum can then act as a valuable source of ideas which teachers can use as a springboard to develop a well-integrated plan of intervention in concert with the child's treatment for the specific handicap.

The *Portage Guide to Early Education* has now been translated into 12 languages and used with a great variety of children in many types of programs. It is important to emphasize three points. First, the guide is not a recipe book for accelerated development or a cure for handicapping conditions, but rather it is a teacher guide and support system to help discover in an organized manner what skills a child has acquired, what skills can appropriately be taught next, and some ways of teaching the chosen skills. Second, individual skills or behaviors may need to be broken down into finer steps, combined or eliminated. Each child will need a different progression of steps based on ability. Third, the success of the guide has been due, in part, to its adaptation to local cultural values and children's and parents' needs. A document such as this needs to be constantly adapted, updated and molded to conform to the context of its use and the needs of the client population.

The Checklist is typically administered at the end of the program year to verify the skills achieved. Program users are also encouraged to re-administer the Checklist periodically to see if previous skills have been maintained or if related skills that have not been directly taught have been acquired.

Activity charts
Once a goal is selected, it is divided into subgoals which serve as weekly instructional objectives. These objectives, along with the directions and materials needed to teach the skill, are written on an activity chart (Fig. 3). Parents can refer to it during the week, and see their child's progress. As parents become familiar with the program and gain confidence in their teaching ability, the number of charts is increased to three to four per week. Charts are written in several developmental areas so that the child receives a complete and integral program. The number of activities may vary, depending upon parental time constraints and willingness to participate in the program.

Home teaching process
Possible objectives should be discussed with the parents and explored with the child to check for appropriateness prior to the visit in which the activity chart is presented. Once the objectives have been agreed upon, the teacher develops an activity chart that takes into account the progress that the child can make in a week

of instruction, and the parents' familiarity with the program.

The natural teaching/learning interaction between the child and parent has been the central point of attention of the Portage Model. The rôle of the home visitor is to facilitate this process and to transfer to the parent sound interactive procedures that can be used after the visitor has left. The focus, though it may initially appear to be on the child, is on the interaction between parent and child. So the home visitor is at the same time a preschool teacher as well as an adult educator.

The Portage Project has developed a four-step process to help parents.

1. *Demonstration and baseline:*
(a) the teacher records the child's pre-instruction responses to the task. This is called the baseline, and provides information on the appropriateness of the selected activity. If the task is too difficult or if the child already knows the skill, the presentation allows the teacher to modify the activity before leaving it with the parents for the week.
(b) after collecting baseline data the home visitor demonstrates the entire activity to the parents. This demonstration provides the parents with a model of the activity, thus making the directions and teaching strategies easier to understand. The demonstration also helps to establish the visitor's credibility as a competent early childhood intervention specialist interested in actually working with the child. For parents who may have had little previous experience with young children or who are non-reading, this demonstration takes on even greater importance.

2. *Modeling:* the parents model the activity for the home visitor. This step provides the parents with an opportunity to practise the activity, and allows the home visitor to see if the parents have understood how to carry it out. The visitor can also give the parents encouragement, praise and additional guidance.

3. *Review:* the parents and home visitor discuss the activity's purpose: when it could most naturally be carried out during the day, what additional household materials could be used to teach or enhance the activity, and how the activity fits into the sequence of instructional goals that will lead to the attainment of long-term goals stated in the IEP. After parents have observed an activity and have had the opportunity to practise, they usually have a number of questions and may also have suggestions on how to modify the activity or how to develop additional activities.

4. *Post baseline:* at the beginning of the subsequent visit the home visitor re-administers the previous week's activities to determine if the instructional objectives have been reached. If not, the teacher modifies the activity or changes the materials. It is essential that objectives are selected and activities so structured that weekly progress is made. It is this progress that maintains parental involvement during the program year. If the activity was successful, the home visitor would typically comment on how well the parents and child are doing, underlining the parents' rôle in their child's success, and proceed to the coming

week's activities.

The four steps of the home teaching process are designed to help children and adults. The first step, demonstration and baseline, provides a concrete reference point for the parents that is directly related to their daily experience in their home environment. The parent modeling step gives immediate feedback on how well the parents have understood the activity and an opportunity for reinforcement and additional guidelines. The review step provides an opportunity for parents to ask questions and give suggestions, thus becoming personally involved in the planning process. And finally, the post baseline step provides an external validation of the parents' work and achievement in teaching their child.

Some time is set aside for informal activities. These are unstructured and used to introduce new materials or objectives that may be used in future weeks. This time can also be used to check previously learned skills or to encourage generalization of a skill to new situations or materials. The tone during this time is playful and game-like to demonstrate that play can serve a very important developmental purpose.

Finally the home visitor discusses any questions, concerns, or problems that the parents may be having. Additional resource material may be brought in or the possibilities of making a referral to a social service agency may be discussed. Often the home teacher will employ formal problem-solving strategies, such as specifying the problem, listing desired outcomes, identifying resources, brainstorming possible solutions, and developing action steps with the parents to address a particular problem. Although not an expert in all fields, the home visitor can be a valuable support to a family with a special-needs child. The entire home visit provides a context for establishing a trusting relationship between the caregiver or parent and the home visitor over a common interest—the optimal development of the child.

During the week between home visits the parents work with the child and record daily progress. The amount of time parents spend working on activities varies greatly depending upon the type of activity, the amount of time the parents have available, and the attention span of the child. It ranges from 15 to 45 minutes daily. Parents are encouraged to work on skills at times when they would most naturally be used: feeding skills during mealtime and undressing skills before going to bed. The intent is not to overburden parents in their already busy schedule but to improve the quality of interaction and instruction in the time that is normally available for caring for the child.

Responsibilities of the home visitor

The home visitor with a full caseload sees 10 to 15 families per week. Home visits range from 60 to 90 minutes each. The home visitor may have additional responsibilities, such as accompanying families on clinic visits, or periodic evaluations of the child and screening other children for possible inclusion into the program. Visitors also attend a weekly half-day staff meeting to review the previous week's work, plan the coming week's activities, meet their supervisor, and discuss problems that have arisen. Periodically professionals from related community resources or speakers on specific topics participate in the staffing to keep staff up to date with what is available in their community and on new developments in the field.

Conclusion

The Model has now been implemented in over 20 countries. The hallmark of successful replications and adaptations has been the simultaneous strict adherence to the principles of the Model and the willingness to adapt specific procedures to the needs of parents and children. Attention to factors such as the experience and educational background of staff, local child-rearing practices, traditional values, family rôles and community involvement in the planning and execution of the program have often been extremely important. Above all the factors has been the careful data-based decision-making process, worked out with parents, on what will best serve the child and facilitate development.

The Portage Project's experience has shown that programs that directly involve parents and caregivers in the education and treatment of their children are feasible, cost-effective, and capable of significantly influencing the child's development and the interaction of parent and child.

REFERENCES

Alpern, G., Boll, T., Shearer, M. S. (1980) *Developmental Profile II.* Aspen, Co.: Psychological Development Publications.

Bluma, S., Shearer, M. S., Frohman, A., Hilliard, J. (1976) *Portage Guide to Early Education.* Portage, Wi.: Cooperative Educational Service Agency No. 12.

Cameron, R. J. (Ed.) (1982) *Working Together: Portage in the U.K.* Windsor, England: NFER—Nelson Publishing Company.

Fredericks, H. D., Baldwin, V., Grove, D. (1976) 'A home-center based parent training model.' *In:* Lillie, D., Trohanis, P. (Eds.) *Teaching Parents to Teach.* N.Y.: Walker Publications.

Jesien, G. (1983) *Preschool Intervention Programs in Developing Countries: Why—And One Example of How.* Portage, Wi.: Cooperative Educational Service Agency No. 12. (Unpublished manuscript.)

—— Aliaga, J., Llanos, M. (1979) 'Validation of the Portage Model in Peru.' *Paper presented at the InterAmerican Congress of Psychology, Lima, Peru.*

Klaus, R. A., Gray, S. W. (1968) 'The early training project for disadvantaged children: a report after five years.' *Monographs of the Society for Research in Child Development,* **33,** No. 120.

McCarthy, D. (1972) *McCarthy Scales of Children's Abilities.* New York: Psychological Corporation.

Peniston, E. (1972) *An Evaluation of the Portage Project.* Portage, Wi.: Cooperative Educational Service Agency No. 12. (Unpublished manuscript.)

Portage Project (1975) 'A home approach to the early education of handicapped children in a rural area.' *Paper presented to the Joint Dissemination Review Panel, U.S.O.E. Washington D.C.*

Revill, S., Blunden, R. (1979) 'A home training service for preschool developmentally handicapped children.' *Behavior Research and Therapy,* **173,** vol. IX, 207–215.

Schortinghuis, N., Frohman, A. (1974) 'A comparison of paraprofessional and professional success with preschool children.' *Journal of Learning Disabilities,* **7.**

Shearer, M. S. (1984) *The Portage Project: a Home-based Early Intervention Model.* Seattle: Educational Service District No. 121.

—— Shearer, D. (1972) 'The Portage Project: a model for early education.' *Exceptional Children,* **39,** 210–217.

Shearer, D., Shearer, M. S. (1976) 'The Portage Project: a model for early childhood intervention.' *In:* Tjossem, T. D. (Ed.) *Intervention Strategies for High Risk Infants and Young Children.* Baltimore: University Park Press. pp. 335–350.

Smith, J., Kushlick, A., Glossop, C. (1977) 'The Wessex Portage Project: a home teaching service for families with a preschool mentally handicapped child.' *Research Report No. 125.* (Available from Health Care Evaluation Research Team, Dawn House, Sleepers Hill, Winchester, Hampshire.)

Thorburn, M. J. (1981) 'In Jamaica, community aides for disabled preschool children.' *Assignment Children,* **53/54,** 117–135. (UNICEF.)

FURTHER READING

Boyd, R. D., Stauber, K. A., Bluma, S. M. (1977) *Instructors Manual: Portage Parent Program.* Portage, Wi.: Cooperative Educational Service Agency No. 12.

Bricker, D., Casuso, V. (1979) 'Family involvement: a critical component of early intervention.' *Exceptional Children,* **46,** 108–116.

Bricker, W. A., Macke, P. R., Levin, J. A., Campbell, P. H. (1981) 'The modifiability of intelligent behavior.' *Journal of Special Education,* **15,** 145–163.

Bronfenbrenner, U. (1975) *A Report on Longitudinal Evaluations of Preschool Programs. Vol. 2: Is Early Intervention Effective?* Washington, D.C.: Department of Health, Education and Welfare, DHEW Publication No. (OHD) 74–25.

Dussault, W. (1982) 'The advocacy process.' *In:* Peters, M., Haring, N. (Eds.) *Building an Alliance for Children: Parents and Professionals.* Seattle: Program Development Assistance System.

Frohman, A. H., Wollenburg, K. (1983) *Get a Jump on Kindergarten: a Handbook for Parents.* Portage, Wi.: Cooperative Educational Service Agency No. 12.

Goldstein, S., Turnbull, A. P. (1982) 'The use of two strategies to increase parent participation in the IEP conference.' *Exceptional Children,* **48** (4), 360–361.

Johnson, N. M., Jens, K. G., Gallagher, R. J., Anderson, J. D. (1980) 'Cognition and effect in infancy: implications for the handicapped.' *New Directions for Exceptional Children,* **3,** 21–36.

Moore, M., Fredericks, H., Baldwin, V. (1981) 'The long-range effects of early childhood education on a trainable mentally retarded population.' *Journal of the Division for Early Childhood,* **4,** 93–110.

Pattison, B. J. (1982) 'The early years and now: the history of the parent advocacy movement.' *In:* Peters, M., Haring, N. (Eds.) *Building an Alliance for Children: Parents and Professionals.* Seattle: Program Development Assistance System.

Ramey, C., Beckman-Bell, P., Gowen, J. W. (1980) 'Infant characteristics and infant-caregiver interactions.' *In:* Gallagher, J. J. (Ed.) *New Directions for Exceptional Children: Parents and Families of Handicapped Children.* San Francisco: Jossey-Bass.

Shearer, M. S. (1976) 'A home-based parent training model.' *In:* Lillie, D., Trohanis, P. (Eds.) *Teaching Parents to Teach.* N.Y.: Walker Publications. pp. 131–148.

Tjossem, T. (Ed.) (1976) *Intervention Strategies for High Risk Infants and Young Children.* Baltimore: University Park Press.

Wolf, B., Griffin, M., Zeger, J., Herwig, J. (1982) *TEACH Training Guide: Development and Implementation of the Individual Services Plan in Head Start.* Portage, Wi.: Cooperative Educational Service Agency No. 12.

4
AIM-ORIENTED MANAGEMENT

David Scrutton

The treatment dilemma

There are patients with cerebral palsy whose treatment is straightforward, simple and finite, but the majority present with a complex developmental disability set within a troubled family and for them the treatment situation is seldom clear-cut. All too frequently a precise prognosis can only be guessed, and yet the treatment (certainly after the first year of life) must increasingly relate to the child's ultimate potential. Any treatment regime may curtail his freedom to some extent and so remove him from the normal world, yet without such help he may not function to his best advantage as an adult.

Some families cannot accept certain treatments: always wanting to do more, or finding even the most limited attendance or treatment too onerous. Some children co-operate and enjoy treatment, others are practically unapproachable; some are at home all day, others at a day nursery or school. Each of these factors affects the possibilities of treatment. So, from the outset, rather than there being a specific treatment for each disorder, there is a treatment for an individual child in his particular circumstances.

There are many treatments for children with cerebral palsy, nearly all needing prolonged clinical experience to be used skilfully and appropriately. No clinic could have the facilities or experience to use them all. Ideally, every therapist treating a cerebral-palsy child should be well trained and have broad experience. In reality this is seldom so for, unlike many less complex (but equally disabling) diseases, there is a need to see very many children with cerebral palsy and watch them grow into adults before it is possible to appreciate the natural history of the disorder and its response to treatment. The almost infinite variety of cerebral palsy (and the lack of a common language to describe this variety accurately) makes learning about it very difficult indeed. Personal experience is the only effective teacher but the incidence of cerebral palsy is too small for experience to be easy to come by and as a result many children are treated by those with insufficient understanding of their problems. It seems to be essential that this group of disorders be *supervised* by those who see the disabled from a large population, probably not less than a million, so that they can build up experience of managing the wide variety of problems presenting at all ages*.

Inevitably, clinics develop an expertise in certain treatments, together with areas of total ignorance and incapacity. For instance, very few clinics have therapists trained in more than one treatment technique or can offer the full range of equipment and modifications to wheelchairs, housing and so on, that many of

---

*This applies equally to therapists, physicians, surgeons and teachers.

the more severely handicapped patients need. The majority of children are lucky to get even one or two items of equipment which are truly specific to their needs and are modified appropriately as they develop. Few children have the possibility of the 'best' treatment. There is too much which *could* be done for some children and, if attempted, it would dominate their lives, together with those of their parents and siblings. Unless a child is removed from his family, or his whole family diverted to his advancement, treatment must become a compromise.

Thus for each aspect of the disorder which might be treated, the therapist should have assessed the prognosis with and without treatment and whether the difference is likely to be significant to the child. The next decision is whether the time needed (by the child and his family) for treatment and travel makes this physically significant effect of *over-all* benefit to him. For time is not on his side: childhood is limited by growth and cannot be extended arbitrarily for therapeutic convenience.

The treatment dilemma is first of all *whether* and *what* to treat; not *how* to do so.

Treatment, no treatment and review

There is a danger inherent in any treatment, whose efficacy is uncertain, being applied to a disorder that cannot be cured. Once it has been decided that treatment should start, it is difficult to find a reason for stopping; yet inevitably the child and his circumstances are changing, for that is the nature of childhood. It is not hard to convince oneself that if this change is for the better then the effective treatment should continue; and if for the worse, then further treatment is essential. Yet as the child is changing, so are his needs. A treatment regime which was ideal six months ago may be a gross intrusion today: then, to improve emerging gait may have been a reasonable aim but now, when he is running about, treatment to this end may serve only to impede his social development.

Thus, treatment needs to be justified before it is started, have precise aims and a review date; and all this should be clearly understood by the parents.

The decision not to treat is a positive one which needs careful discussion with the parents. It must be seen to be a reasonable response to their child's needs, and not as indifference or neglect. This decision too requires review.

From treatment to management

The skilled handling of cerebral-palsy infants and children by therapists can be impressive to watch and the immediate effects obvious and dramatic. Such treatments, accompanied by confidently stated long-term aims, are persuasive and hard to contest. However, experience has led me to consider that however good the immediate effect, the carry-over into out-of-treament life is often small (particularly after the first year of life) and the long-term outcome by no means so impressive.

Clinical experience points to the conclusion that the effective parts of a treatment are those which become part of the child's life: a comparatively small (but carefully selected) therapy input then has a significant effect. Consequently, treatment sessions become training sessions for parents and care staff and, since the physical management has to be relevant to the child's day, it is best if these are at home, day nursery or school, rather than the child attending the hospital. Of course such an approach to treatment is not original. However, it was not adopted as a copy of an existing system, but as an individual response to clinical experience. It involves far more than advice to parents on play, bathing, feeding, positioning and exercises. It is not a decision to avoid the use of more formal treatment techniques—such as muscle strengthening, orthotics and plastering. It is a deliberate shift of emphasis from solely hospital-oriented criteria for action towards the broader social, educational and family-based criteria, with the consideration that a treatment which may be ideal for a child in one circumstance may be totally inappropriate in other circumstances. Yet such a system—often referred to as 'management'—is difficult to present. There is no treatment room with equipment or full waiting-room, and usually there are no dramatic in-treatment improvements to demonstrate. In short, there is no system to the treatment itself, for the system, if any, is in the criteria for deciding treatment aims and priorities.

As far as I can tell, it seems to be at least as effective and frequently more effective than treatment approaches which are manifestly more skilful. Moreover, I get the impression that the child has greater scope to develop as a person and the parents have the opportunity for a more realistic view of their child and situation.

Management and the therapist
However, management techniques are harder to teach and give much less support to the inexperienced therapist's morale. Cerebral palsy is a very confusing and unsettling disorder to deal with on a day-to-day basis and it is reassuring to know that one is part of a respectably established group of like-minded colleagues and obviously using skilled therapy techniques. For it is not comfortable to step outside the treatment room and face the child's and family's real problems alone. One reason for this deserves discussion. In the abstract one can analyse a clinical problem, arrive at a view and decide on aims and means; but this is quite different from ensuring parental acceptance and co-operation day after day. Quite simply, it is extremely difficult to prevent the treatment from appearing over-simple and parents and care staff often require some proof of expertise. It demands a clear-sighted determination to bear up under this assault and many therapists prefer to adopt an accepted approach which provides personal security together with a ready-made series and variety of exercises, each allowing a seemingly logical transition to the next stage of treatment.

Those who are not involved in building and sustaining such a relationship with the anxious parents of a handicapped child probably consider such a ploy both unnecessary and inexcusable, but I find it hard to agree. However much a 'method' attitude to treatment may infuriate me at times, I have great sympathy for it and if we wish to have enough therapists willing to work with these families we must find ways of working which attract and retain them. For have no doubt, most of these children will be treated in some way by someone—their parents will see to that. Above all, we need to devise a framework, flexible enough to meet the needs of both children and parents, which allows us to offer the children the physical management most appropriate to their needs. It may be that a 'method' approach, with all the limitations inherent in such a concept, will prove the best way to do this for most clinics, most therapists, most children and most families.

The essential difference between a management approach and treatment
It is not easy to state 'this is treatment, that is management'. Nevertheless, the differences are real; fundamentally they are differences of attitude.

Treatment usually happens in a hospital or clinic and works on an out-patient system. The therapist is on her territory, the child and parents are the visitors. It is inherent in management that it is the parents and child who are at home and the therapist must fit in to their lifestyle and their timetable.

Treatment is exercise-oriented; if an exercise is correct for a child, and the parents are to do it at home, then that is the exercise they do. Whereas a management approach would be aim-oriented, seeking out how this family, with all its skills and limitations, can achieve this or that end.

Treatment is therapist-oriented, it is her skills which are paramount. Management, however, sees the therapist as the adviser and catalyst for the therapeutic attitudes and actions of the parents. The parents claim all the successes but only in such a way that they do not feel responsible for the failures.

Treatment may include home management advice, but it is secondary to the therapist's treatment; whereas any skilled precise techniques taught to the parents as part of their child's management are seen as part of the management, not as superseding it.

Treatment can be given without visiting the child's home, because it is disorder-oriented. On the other hand, management can hardly be undertaken without a good understanding of the home and the family's advantages and limitations. It is essentially family- or situation-oriented.

Aim-oriented management
From the above it may be seen that giving some advice on handling a child at home or teaching the parents skilled exercises for their child do not represent what is meant here by 'management', though they are a recognition that the therapist is not supreme. Equally it must be emphasised that management cannot always fulfil all therapeutic needs of the child and there are times when the parents or care staff, however well-intentioned, are no substitute for the therapist's skilled treatment.

Therapy for cerebral palsy therefore requires several essential features:
(1) The most accurate possible prognosis (not only locomotor).
(2) A list of problems.
(3) An assessment of which problems can be eliminated or ameliorated.
(4) An assessment of the child's situation, for instance:
    (a) Where is he during the day? When could therapy occur? What co-operation is likely from the child, the parents, the teachers, or care staff?
    (b) Would therapy interrupt other activities? How important are these? Is therapy of overriding importance? Could it be arranged so as to improve the other activities?

(c) At night: does he sleep well? Would he tolerate night splinting or positioning?

(5) From this over-all assessment a list of practical aims and means of therapy can be made and given a priority.

(6) This is discussed with the child, the parents and all those involved so that agreement can be reached on the aims and means, together with a review date.

Thus it is impossible to write about how one would manage a child with a specific problem, let alone a particular diagnosis. However, without being more detailed it might be difficult for the reader to have an idea of the kind of things that might be done. Perhaps the most concise way of dealing with this is to give some examples, bearing in mind that they are examples of how a child could be managed, rather than should be or would be managed.

Example 1

Problem: Consistent preferred head turning (PHT) and asymmetric tonic neck response (ATNR) in an infant with quadriplegic cerebral palsy—probably rigid/dystonic.

Consideration: Persisting head turning (Robson 1968) if retained has disastrous effects (Fulford and Brown 1976), particularly when associated with a strong ATNR. We cannot treat the ATNR as such—it will diminish or remain depending on factors within the child. We can usually prevent the PHT and ATNR from being perfected through practice—leading to unnecessarily retained asymmetry long after the response has disappeared—and so reduce the effect this has on gross movement and posture.

Aim: To encourage head turning to the opposite side and movements and postures against the asymmetric response.

Action:

(1) Parents to approach, play and feed the child from the opposite side.

(2) Use a foam cut-out to hold his head to the neutral or opposite side when supine or in a 'baby relax'.

(3) Use a prone wedge: some infants lose all preferred head turning in a supported prone position, others spontaneously turn to the opposite side.

(4) Corner seat: placed high in the room (on a table) to encourage looking down and positioned so that the preferred side is to a blank wall. Preferred head turning is often less in sitting than supine.

(5) Supported sitting propping on an extended 'occipital' arm.

(6) Creeping: facilitating jaw-side leg flexion and abduction followed by symmetrical creeping facilitated through shoulder girdle or head/neck.

(7) Jaw-side upper limb exploring face, sucking fingers, *etc.*

(8) Any symmetrical activity.

Example 2: between-heel sitting

Many therapists strongly advise parents of any cerebral-palsy child liable to femoral neck anteversion (and internal rotation gait) not to allow him to sit between heels. The following points are worth noting:

(1) Between-heel sitting is the preferred sitting posture of many normal children, tends to run in families and causes them no problems.

(2) The ranges of hip internal and external rotation in flexion (the sitting posture) and extension (the standing/walking position which is of concern) are frequently unrelated. Many cerebral-palsy children with nil external rotation in extension have 40 degrees or so external rotation in flexion.

(3) Sitting between heels is very uncomfortable unless one *already has* sufficient internal rotation to allow the buttocks to rest on the floor. Other children do not choose it.

(4) The alternative postures suggested are usually very difficult for the confirmed between-heel sitter with a motor disorder, and in cerebral palsy lead to a backward rotation of the pelvis, kyphotic spine, poking chin, and difficulty with hand function because of the unstable base.

(5) Between-heel sitting, for those who prefer it, gives a very stable base, aligns the pelvis for good spinal posture and head control and frees the hands for use.

(6) Many families have been exasperated by the day-in day-out battle to prevent their child doing something which is natural, efficient and ideal in all respects except (perhaps) one.

Between-heel sitting offers far more advantages than disadvantages to nearly all children with spastic diplegia or athetosis.

Example 3
Problem: To promote symmetrical gait in an infant with hemiplegia.
Consideration: Unless there is another major handicap, all children with infantile hemiplegic cerebral palsy walk, and usually not very much later than comparable normal children. Unlike the upper limb, we know the child will use the leg and the problem is how it is used.
Aims: Discourage foot/ankle fixed deformity and ensure a plantigrade foot and a level pelvis.
Action:
(1) Stretching the tendo achilles and gastrocnemius daily. I am not convinced that passive stretching prevents fixed deformity, but most parents will do this passive movement anyway and so should be taught to do it properly. Persistent ankle/foot mobile deformity may require night splinting which is usually well tolerated by an infant.

(2) Encourage the infant to kick both legs in the bath. Avoid using a bouncer, sit-in baby walker or any supported standing (on a lap, for instance) with the leg used only as a stiff prop.

(3) Once the child can sit, practise getting to standing through half-kneeling pushing up (and lowering) on the hemiplegic leg. Practise standing on the hemiplegic leg only, playing at a table—the other leg can be flexed at the knee and held between one's legs when kneeling behind the child.

(4) As soon as he spontaneously gets to standing, he must have a plantigrade foot and equality of leg length which may require an orthosis (I prefer a polypropelene AFO) and a shoe raise. Unless the fixed point of the leg (the weight-bearing foot) is

54

dynamically stable, the whole body will be forced into asymmetric compensatory postures.

(5) When walking with an adult, hold the hemiplegic hand to prevent that side of the body lagging behind.

(6) Not all hemiplegic gait is identical. There are two major types: those who semiflex the hip and knee, and those who hyperextend the knee. The role of an AFO will be different for each (Scrutton 1976).

Example 4

Problem: Day-to-day posture of a severe quadriplegic cerebral-palsy child of whatever type without any secure postural ability.

Consideration: Such a child needs a variety of postures, partly because he cannot be expected to remain in one position all day, but also to give him a variety of opportunities and experiences. The child needs positions in which (i) he can best function, (ii) allow him to learn to hold the posture himself, (iii) he is most easily cared for (*e.g.* fed), and (iv) he can be comfortable. These aims may conflict and a chair for learning head or trunk control (say) may be useless for learning to type, *etc.* Sitting assumes great importance simply because it is the best compromise, allowing activity and mobility, without necessarily requiring good postural ability.

Aim: To allow a number of postures for comfort, variety and to prevent deformity. To promote function (including mobility). To promote the learning of postural ability.

Action:

Prone lying over a wedge-shaped foam cushion promotes head control, arm support and back extension.

Side lying is a good position for bimanual mid-line play with the head firmly supported. Correction of postural lateral spinal curvature over a fixed pad is possible.

Sitting on the floor in a corner seat. These must be made for the individual size and needs of the child. The height of the backrest, size of the pommel, height and size of the tray vary greatly from child to child. A child with very tight hamstrings is unlikely to stretch them in this position and will tend to flex the knees or rotate the pelvis.

Chair sitting. Fundamental to sitting is a correctly positioned and stable pelvis; without this, sitting inevitably becomes 'upright lying'. This requires correct chair depth, width and height to foot rest: only then can consideration be given to how the trunk is to be positioned and supported. The exception to this is when severe fixed deformity would cause the shoulders to be in a position such that head control would be impossible, or head position impractical. Then, and perhaps only then, seating is from the head downwards.

Upright kneeling is useful to get weight-bearing through the hips when knee or ankle/foot deformity prevents supported standing. It is easily achieved in a standing frame with minimal modification and has the advantages of preventing mass extension, allowing greater hip abduction (by relaxing the medial hamstrings) and giving good control of hip rotation.

Standing. Supported standing in a Flexistand or prone stander allows a radical change of posture and orientation, fully extends the hips and knees and usually gives a better balance of activity between the flexor and extensor muscle groups.

Example 5

Problem: Asymmetric hip deformity—windswept hips.

Consideration: Everything possible should be done to oppose the habitual adoption of an asymmetric hip posture as it frequently leads to dislocation of the adducted and internally rotated hip and to scoliosis. What starts in infancy as an apparently benign tendency can become the single most important factor in the adolescent's and adult's life, leading to continual pain or discomfort and difficulty in nursing care. It is likely that early persistent postural management can significantly alter the outcome. It is interesting that dislocation seldom occurs (i) subsequent to a child walking (although this might be no more than a reflection of the severity of the disorder), (ii) in previously normal children who have walked and subsequently suffer brain insult, regardless of the degree and persistence of windsweeping, (iii) in the abducted hip in spite of the unbalanced muscle activity (except after adductor tenotomy when it can dislocate anteriorly). Scoliosis is usually secondary to the pelvic asymmetry. For these children pelvic symmetry seems important in preventing scoliosis, and the factors in preventing dislocation are (i) abduction and external rotation, and (ii) early weight-bearing.

Aims: To encourage symmetrical posture (sometimes by practising the opposite asymmetry).

Action:

(1) See 'Action' for Example 1.

(2) In prone on a wedge-tie the ankle of the 'adducted' leg to the opposite knee, thus holding the hip in abduction and external rotation.

(3) Sit with the 'adducted' hip held in abduction by firmly locating the pelvis (abducting that leg without locating the pelvis succeeds only in rotating the pelvis). For a method of fixation see Scrutton 1978.

(4) Standing: early weight-bearing through the hips, preferably in standing but in upright kneeling if knee or foot deformity dictates. A sit-in baby walker and 'baby bouncer' are to be avoided as weight-bearing is intermittent only and usually in the position of deformity. I prefer a standing frame, but children who cannot cope with one can use a prone stander. The 'adducted' hip should be abducted and externally rotated.

(5) Parents should be shown how to discourage the windswept posture at all times.

(6) Sleeping: if the knees are semiflexed, children without fixed deformity can sleep windswept to the opposite side, held there by a well tucked-in drawsheet over the legs only.

Example 6

Problem: An educable school-aged child with severe quadriplegic athetosis.

Consideration: I have never found any physical treatment which reduces athetosis. However, involuntary movements are usually at a minimum when the child is (i) well supported, (ii) emotionally secure and (iii) attempting a purposeful movement which has an outcome he desires and which he knows he can achieve. Severe involuntary movement combined with hypertonus nearly always leads to fixed and structural deformity and it is obvious that these should be discouraged, particularly at the hips and spine. Seldom, if ever, should any physical treatment aim be allowed to interfere significantly with the (intelligent) child learning a means of communication.

Aims:

(1) To create physical circumstances in which he can learn to communicate—probably the most important aim.

(2) To provide a means of mobility.

(3) To give experience of functional movement (which will require a stable postural background).

(4) To give opportunity to experience and practise postural stability from which functional voluntary movement may be possible.

Conclusion

These few examples inevitably give a limited and unbalanced view of what is really involved. Fundamentally I do not think that enough is known of the neuropathology, the various responses of the different types of cerebral palsy to treatment, the effects of those treatments, the mechanisms producing fixed deformity or the true nature and influence of patterns of locomotor development. Consequently it seems unwarranted to base a treatment upon them.

However, we do have some understanding of the natural history of these disorders and so can help the child to avoid most of the more common pitfalls. We also have experience of the problems these children present their families. Thus the management approach is concerned with the practical problems facing the child and those caring for him.

There are three fundamental aims governing intervention:

(1) To reduce the handicapping effect of the disorder. For instance, to improve movement and posture, prevent or reduce deformity, and create circumstances in which the child can experience and understand his environment better.

(2) To promote the child's assets. Handicapped people are all too easily seen as the sum of their deficits, an aggregation of problems which need treatment, and the real person is obscured by this facade. Intervention aimed at reducing handicap must not interfere with the nurturing of any assets. Each single ability has disproportionate significance in the life of a disabled person.

(3) To support the family, tailoring the intervention to suit their needs as well as the child's.

These aims are subservient to one overriding aim: an endeavour to guide the child towards adulthood with a purpose in life and with the best possibility of fulfilling himself.

REFERENCES

Fulford, G. E., Brown, J. K. (1976) 'Position as a cause of deformity in children with cerebral palsy.' *Developmental Medicine and Child Neurology*, **18**, 305–314.

Robson, P. (1968) 'Persisting head turning in the early months: some effects in the early years.' *Developmental Medicine and Child Neurology*, **10**, 82–92.

Scrutton, D. R. (1976) 'The physical management of children with hemiplegia.' *Physiotherapy*, **62**, 285–293.

—— (1978) 'Developmental deformity and the profoundly retarded child.' *In:* Apley, J. (Ed.) *The Care of the Handicapped Child*. London: S.I.M.P. with Heinemann; Philadelphia: Lippincott.

5

WINTHROP PHELPS AND THE CHILDREN'S REHABILITATION INSTITUTE

Anita H. Slominski

Introduction

Dr. Winthrop Morgan Phelps devoted his medical career to the development of treatment for the cerebral-palsied child, and to the training of physicians and therapists to give that treatment. He influenced countless professional people throughout the world, and is considered by many to have been the first person to develop a coherent and systematic approach to treatment. Much of his teaching is still current in some form today, and often goes unattributed since it is so fundamental. For example, active motion and stimulation activities, to prevent contractures and to awaken the interest of even the most severely disabled children to some form of purposeful play, are as popular today as when he first prescribed them. He warned against over-protection and stressed the need for active independence; and he recommended the concept of individual testing and assessment so that a realistic comprehensive program could be developed. He also believed every child would progress through each stage of normal physical development (head control, sitting, crawling and so forth) and that he could speed that development with therapy or special equipment— 'positioning to function' or positioning to develop a motor pattern (Phelps and Hopkins 1958, Slominski and Hamant 1971).

As an orthopedic resident in 1923, Phelps became inspired by the work of Bronson Crothers, a pediatric neurologist who was exploring new theories of treatment at Boston Children's Hospital (Samilson 1975). Reviewing the empirical work begun in 1891 by Miss Jennie Colby, a gymnast, and expanded by Mary E. Trainor RPT (one of the very first graduates from a physical therapy school, and the then director of the Clinic for Muscle Training of Paralytic Cases), both Phelps and Crothers were impressed with the success of children's rhymes used with remedial exercises to develop strength or skill in a weakened muscle or impaired muscle-group (Egel 1948, Jones 1967). These women trainers believed that some children had normal mentality behind a mask of dyskinesia (uncontrolled motion) and that they would co-operate and learn. Parents were taught these exercises to do at home a specified number of times daily, with monthly or bi-monthly reviews with the therapist. In this specialized clinic a total program was emphasized for the evolving child. Crothers and Phelps expanded the team effort to include psychological evaluations in program planning. Their pioneering research brought in Elizabeth E. Lord from Boston Children's Hospital, and Edgar H. Doll from the Training School at Vineland, New Jersey (Lord 1937). Together they found that even extreme cases of motor disability did not necessarily eliminate normal mentality: normal intelligence could exist in children with dyskinetic problems. Phelps adopted the term 'cerebral palsy' to separate those children with normal intelligence and a motor/sensory problem from those with mental retardation (Crother 1959, Brunyate 1963). He further explained that a non-progressive lesion in the brain could be associated with any combination of abnormalities, including sensory or mental deviations, visual or auditory losses, seizures and motor deficiencies, as he separated those of cerebral origin from those originating from damage of the spinal cord (polio) or the peripheral nervous system (Phelps 1952). He thought that the complex problems associated with cerebral palsy necessitated expanding the multidisciplinary team even further; that information should be shared with all team members before designing a specific program for a child; and that the combined plan should be shared with the parents (Jones 1967).

It was necessary to train such specialists to work together, to collaborate and to trust each other to work for a common goal. In 1936 he resigned as director of orthopedics at the Yale School of Medicine, and established the residential center for children and staff training at the Children's Rehabilitation Institute (CRI) in Cockeysville, Maryland. Continuing his work as orthopedic consultant for children with cerebral palsy throughout the States and abroad, he drew students from all parts of the world to his training center; many of these students later developed programs of their own on their home fronts.

In 1944, through the Easter Seal Society/National Society for Crippled Children and Adults, he published and circulated the pamphlet *The Farthest Corner—an Outline for the Cerebral Palsy Problem* (4th edition 1947). By 1946 the Society had decided it needed a Cerebral Palsy Division, and Dr. Phelps brought together physician specialists with strong interests in cerebral palsy: Bronson Crothers the pediatric neurologist, George Deaver the physiatrist, neurophysiologist Temple Fay, the internist Earl Carlson, and Meyer Perlstein the pediatrician. This small group encouraged nationwide (and international) interest in the handicapped child, which precipitated the formation of the American Academy for Cerebral Palsy, of which Phelps became the first president at the Chicago meeting in 1947 (Scherzer and Tscharnuter 1982). There was now a multispeciality professional organization to promote research and training.

Rationale

The Phelps training program at CRI was based on his view that realistic goals could be established by the team for each child, and that the highest degree of improvement could be obtained with an individually integrated program (Kahmann 1938, Phelps 1941a). He placed great emphasis on differential diagnosis, and disputed the concept that all cerebral-palsied people were spastic. He considered cerebral palsy to be a group of conditions: spasticity, athetosis, ataxia, rigidity and tremor (Phelps 1949, Fay 1950, Denhoff and Robinault 1960).

Consequently many different types of treatment were used: massage, passive motion, active assisted motion, active motion, resisted motion, conditioned motion, automatic motion, combined motion, rest, relaxation, motion from a relaxed position, balance, reciprocation, reach and grasp, and the acquisition of various skills (see Appendix I). Individual programs incorporated any or all of these. His team worked with individual muscles, gross movement patterns (Fay 1946, 1954), and with control or inhibition of abnormal motions. Synergistic movements were stimulated by music and rhymes to develop a specific pattern or group of patterns, which could later take place when the rhymes were repeated without the music. This association aided many children in hand-to-mouth patterns for feeding themselves, and reciprocal leg movements for walking.

Visual stimulation with mirrors was often used, as was a metronome. Braces and other orthotic devices were used to help regulate muscle tone and assist postural control so that one extremity could move purposefully by itself (Phelps 1952). He often said, 'All children need rest and relaxation. Rest is freedom from activity; many of my cerebral-palsied children need braces or splints or special furniture just to accomplish rest' (Slominski 1950–54). Each of his team therapists began a patient's treatment from a rest-relaxed position and progressed to purposeful activity.

He considered that 'A person having cerebral palsy is susceptible to retraining which may be compared to training the normal person in skills, such as playing the piano. The amount of retraining possible is extremely variable and dependent on the degree and the areas of damage to the brain, habit, innate skill, and psychological attitude of the individual toward his handicap' (Brunyate 1963). Anyone being taught the piano, or learning to skate or ski, trains various co-ordinated mechanisms involving unusual synergistic control and balance, which are gradually improved and perfected. All treatments designed and prescribed by Phelps were directed to accomplishing motor skills and self-help. He encouraged his therapists to use the Gesell Developmental Scales with children learning motor skills, in the proper order and progressing through all the steps. While every normal child walks sooner or later as an automatic stage of motor development, the child with cerebral palsy has to be taught with repetitive practice.

Phelps believed that physical and mental education should be parallel, and that neither should advance beyond the other. Daily exercise should not be sacrificed for homework time; reading could be done in a standing table; memorizing verse or math tables could be done during reciprocal exercises. It is most important for the child to perceive himself as he does his peers, making normal progress, receiving the same homework and written assignments and being expected to complete his own work, perhaps with the exception of typing rather than writing his lessons. Everyone must do his share and know that he has done his share, exceptions being made only when absolutely necessary.

Goals
Phelps insisted on psychological re-evaluations to assist the team and parents in setting new goals. Expectations that were too high were devastating to the child's self-image, and those with less than normal potential needed more time to achieve a goal. Parents needed help in understanding their child's mental and physical limitations. The psychologist and social worker received cues from the other team members and counselled parents or referred them to parent support groups. Each

therapist must direct the parent toward a realistic goal, help them accept small gains, and understand those that were hard to visualize. Some parents needed to learn alternative ways to teach their child to be more productive. Minor crafts might lead to employment in a sheltered workshop if the person has learned good work habits. Phelps told parents: 'Everyone needs to be productive within their own family whenever possible. Idleness or a feeling of uselessness creates boredom, dissatisfaction and frustration' (Phelps and Hopkins 1958).

Crafts and toys were used to motivate and maintain the child's interest (Carlson 1941). Carlson described occupational therapy as 'one excellent way of arousing the patient's interest' and reported that children who received training in a variety of crafts evidenced a remarkable improvement in muscular control: 'Children [who] soon became bored with their exercises, with moving their muscles simply for the sake of the muscles, delighted in using their hands purposefully and soon had much better control over them.'

Meetings were arranged so that parents could discuss their mutual problems with each other or with a panel of experts. Diet was a favorite topic, since many parents over-indulged their children as a way of showing love (Phelps 1951). He considered over-eating to be one of the greatest problems for spastic children since they do not burn up the extra calories (Phelps and Hopkins 1958).

The Phelps habilitation programs at CRI were set up on a three-month goal plan, followed by two weeks of vacation. This hiatus was a safety-valve for both children and staff. During the vacation period, the children still wore day or night braces and used adapted equipment, but they did not have to do daily exercises (though many parents found devious ways to 'play exercise games').

Treatment goals were reviewed monthly or quarterly as needed, and were upgraded and designed to include all family members, especially siblings. Parents were urged to join and contribute to these sessions. Team communication and co-operation promoted the best over-all plan for each person: each member had a personal investment in the plan and its anticipated goals. Beginning with relaxation, exercising in the planes of normal motion, controlling movement mechanically, and finally reaching normal skeletal alignment, resulted in many children learning to care for themselves, walk, and later become employable (Gillette 1969). And, as recorded by Jones (1967), 'Motor re-education and relaxation were considered to be the most important therapeutic agents now known to be effective for the cerebral palsies'.

Treatment

All treatment began with a modification of Jacobson's progressive relaxation (Jacobson 1938). Sometimes a semi-darkened room was used. Often wrapping and cuddling with a soft blanket and flexing the athetoid child into a fetal position brought about total relaxation. Sandbags, braces or other equipment could be used to hold the child while he 'thought about loosening' his arm. First contracting a muscle or group of muscles, then 'letting go', may be more meaningful to the child than the term 'relax': *e.g.* making a fist with the child's hand for him to maintain, then asking him to let go. Phelps taught that motion from a relaxed position is most important to the athetoid patient, and that moving a hand to grasp a spoon for self-feeding without losing head control could be a goal after total relaxation. This might be followed by passive motion, active assisted motion, active motion and resisted motion (against gravity). Since kinesthetic muscle sense is disturbed in cerebral palsy, exercises and therapy should be done in the gravitational field, not under water as with polio patients. Water may be used for general recreation, and can be useful for training mouth closure and sustaining breath, but it is not a substitute for exercise against gravity. Since reciprocation must be learned by the child with cerebral palsy, conditioned motions were taught with children's songs as the therapists moved the child through the range of desired action (Egel 1948). Conditioning exercises often were assisted with braces or mechanical aids; parallel bars, skis, quad canes or crutches (Phelps 1941*b*, 1942). Walkers were not used, as he taught that they not only eliminated reciprocation of the hips and shoulders, but also produced a lunging gait and greatly delayed independent standing balance (Phelps and Hopkins 1958).

Bracing
Preventative measures were foremost in Phelps's treatment plans. Braces were used to control the limbs. In the growing child with cerebral palsy, muscles pull abnormally against each other, causing contractures in the flexor groups and weakness in the extensor groups. He compared the growing extremities to beans or ivy growing around a pole: a child sitting all day will have the 'twisting ivy' legs, while one using long-leg braces for scheduled standing with knee and hip extension will keep the 'ivy legs' growing straight, tall and not twisted or crooked (Phelps 1952, Phelps and Hopkins 1958). Thus braces were used to support weak muscles, control overactive muscles, stabilize those lacking balance, and to control and prevent scissoring or adduction in the athetoid child whose extensive involuntary motion prevents normal balance. For young children, braces often support weakness so that weight-bearing can take place to develop the hip sockets and distribute the child's weight evenly on both feet. A back and head/neck brace could aid in the control of neck hyperextension, and excessive rotary head motion, so enabling the child to focus his eyes. A collar brace alone will not support the head and prevent neck hyperextension, but a ball-bearing adjustable swivel attached to a head-helmet could limit head rotation. Arm braces or splints might be used for support, control or prevention, just as leg braces were used, or even to assist the development of hand and finger motion. The flailing athetoid child might use them for stabilization, *e.g.* to keep one or both arms on his lap, tray or table. A time schedule for wearing arm braces or splints was part of the treatment plan. This kind of arm stabilization by brace or wrist cuff enabled some children to learn to drink from a glass through a straw.

Sleeping patterns were observed, since braces or splints might be used only at night. Since the child grows during sleep, a position of extreme flexion allows the flexor muscles to remain short and causes contractures. A child unable to turn over independently in bed could develop 'wind-swept' hips, with subluxation on the weaker side. Splints, sandbags, or special wedges were used to prevent these deformities during sleep. Children in bed look towards interesting sounds or activities, so the location of the bed can be important. The team also considered the problem of too much sleep or too long a nap, which might keep the child awake at the wrong time. Parents were also taught how to lift and carry their child correctly, allowing the child to do as much of every body transfer as possible. This teaching also prevented back injuries in the ageing parents (Phelps and Hopkins 1958).

Drugs
Another consideration was the use of muscle relaxants or drugs to control seizures. Documentation of use was carefully recorded by therapists and parents. Phelps did extensive experimental drug research which was helpful to many of his patients (Phelps 1959).

Surgery
Phelps believed there was a right time for surgery. He used serial casting and bracing preoperatively; postoperative bracing and splinting maintained corrections gained surgically. He ensured that parents and children understood the reasons for operating, and discussed the postoperative care in great detail. With him, 'preplanning and understanding was the key to successful therapy' (Phelps 1957, Phelps and Hopkins 1958).

Equipment
Most of today's adaptive equipment can be traced back to Phelps and his staff. For a child lacking head control and trunk balance braces, and special furniture were often used to place him in a stable position so that he could benefit from therapy (Egel 1948, Phelps and Hopkins 1958, Slominski and Hamant 1971). Phelps believed that the children needed to feel safe; since often they lacked sensory awareness in space, they were afraid of falling. Treatment tables were wide and covered with a comfortable mat. Cut-out tables and special lap-trays were fitted to each child's chair or wheelchair to support the elbows and forearms if necessary for table therapy, self-feeding or schoolwork. Chairs were built with a flexed seat to prevent extensor thrust and to provide head support (NSCCA 1950). Corsets and various suspender-type jackets or harness straps were used for trunk balance and stabilization. Only with proper positioning—*i.e.* the child not struggling to sit upright—could energy be preserved: the child could then direct his eyes and mind to the task in hand. Feet were placed flat on the floor or dorsiflexed 10 to 15 degrees on footrests to prevent body thrusting, using ankle-straps or toe-straps to keep them in place. Pelvic or thoracic lateral wings were added to chairs to prevent scoliosis and to help the child sit upright. Abductor cuffs or wedges might be used in sitting to stabilize the athetoid pelvis or to prevent adduction of the thighs of the spastic child or adult. Table-tops might be raised, dropped or tilted to place writing-paper or typewriters at the best possible angle for work. Typewriter keyboard covers were designed to allow a finger or typing stick to drop into the hole and prevent the athetoid hand from striking numerous keys together (Martin 1940, Brunyate 1952). Handle modifications were made to toys, games and eating

utensils as well as pencils and tricycle handlebars. Wooden boards were jigged to hold dishes and cups in one place for athetoid or ataxic children. Each patient's problems were analysed by the whole team, then adaptations or corrected work planes were adjusted to enable the requested task to be performed easily (Miller *et al.* 1955).

Wheelchairs
Parents were expected to consult the therapists about the purchase of wheelchairs or other adapted equipment, and children were encouraged to wheel their own chairs whenever possible. No one was allowed to spend the entire day in a wheelchair.

Daily living
Time schedules included therapy out of the chair, possibly a different chair for feeding or relaxation, and using a standing table, a creeper, crawler or parallel bars. CRI had a full-time carpenter to build and rebuild adapted equipment on prescription from Phelps and his team.

Building plans were sent home with some children who would be using equipment over long periods of time. Room designs or bathroom plans were reviewed by the occupational therapist to provide the best motivation for physical activity. Phelps often commented that grooming and the ability to care for oneself become more important as the person matures. By the age of 11, most children are straining to achieve adult skills: the handicapped child also has these needs, and care must be taken to provide him with the greatest opportunities for success. That is the time to make vocational plans and to set reasonable goals for physical growth and independence. Phelps repeated frequently: 'Too often well-meaning parents and others smother the child with too much assistance and no opportunity to help himself. Parents give the deleterious excuse: "It takes him too long, it's faster if I help him or do it myself". Motivation is destroyed by such attitudes, and complacency like that never lets him know he might have been able to do it alone.'

When a mother learns a seating position for her child that will make it easier to feed him, she is more willing to concentrate on head and mouth control since she does not have to struggle with a wriggling child slipping off her lap (Hadra 1955). Further training in feeding, such as chewing, sucking and variations of food and utensils, can be added as the occupational and speech therapists review progress. These are not to take place at the family meal-time, but are scheduled with a time limit to keep up the motivation of mother and child. Proper conditioning of speech muscles, face and tongue are reviewed. Relaxation and allowing time to complete the requested motion are paramount.

Phelps realised that reaching and grasping require a combination of joint motions, and usually these were taught in a sitting position. Aids might be used to stabilize joints or extremities, especially for the athetoid person. Once voluntary reach grasp and release has been attained, skill training can begin. Skills are taught when joint motions are performed with rhythmical ease. Finger or wrist splints or weighted cuffs were used for control or ease of motion, but any equipment used in this way was considered a training device, to be discarded as soon as the motion or skill could be completed without the artificial aid.

Relaxation chairs were modelled on the Adirondak lawn-chair* and were used alone or in conjunction with body braces to promote a restful posture for athetoid or ataxic patients. Every effort was made to enable them to maintain an upright position without struggling against gravity, so that they could concentrate on eating, schoolwork or recreation.

Hand dominance

After reviewing the family history on hand dominance, the occupational therapist evaluated and recorded the child's abilities and noted which hand, eye or leg was used first. Phelps and others believed that a lack of dominance was sometimes a cause of seizures and behavior problems. He taught that when handicap involved the dominant hand and arm, a shift in dominance must be trained or established. He believed that no behavior problems would appear if this dominance shift takes place before the age of two: if the shift is delayed or does not occur, as more is demanded of the child with maturation, inability to cope with a poorly co-ordinated hand affects his behavior (Doll *et al.* 1951, Price 1954, Brunyate 1963). Using the opposite hand, leg and eye, or crossed dominance, can cause problems with balance and body awareness in space.

Other considerations

Vision and hearing should be re-evaluated on a regular basis: especially often if the child wears appliances. Dental care is also very important. Over-biting or receding jaws were treated as early as possible to provide jaw alignment for chewing, eating and speaking. High palates might also need an orthosis for eating or speaking.

Phelps shared the findings of psychological testing with the parents so that they could make sensible plans for the future care of their child. They needed to know what might be expected rather than to hope for unrealistic achievements and constantly be facing failure and disappointment. His speech therapist, psychologist and others in his team stressed the need for parents to expose the children to good speech: not to slur words or talk too fast, but to speak distinctly and repeat phrases. Parents were asked to read aloud to the child to develop thought progression. Rhymes are good because of their rhythm and repetition. Talking teaches the child to motivate his senses: to smell the rain, to hear the birds, to see the aeroplane, to listen to the cars, to feel the grass, to taste the salt (Phelps and Hopkins 1958).

Mirrors were used by all therapists to help children acquire a visual image in space and to enhance their self-esteem and awareness. In some cases they also helped to control drooling and improve mouth closure. For the very severely handicapped, the team of therapists devised communication boards, which were modified as the child advanced in learning school skills. All aids were designed so

*A rigid wooden slatted chair with sloping seat and back.

that they could be improved upon when proficiency had been demonstrated.

Recreational interests were developed within the person's limits. The plan was for as normal a life as possible, to be enjoyed to its fullest. Again, equipment was used to develop independent skills: book-holders, camera jigs, or record-player adaptations were made with the ingenuity of Phelps's team and his carpenter. Useful sitting toys were made from nail-kegs; sanded or covered with cloth, mounted on small castors and with a wooden animal-head with ears (handles for the child to grasp), these enabled the child to sit in a natural, relaxed abduction position and to move his feet on the floor.

Summary
Dr. Phelps was a rare combination of family physician and specialist, who pulled together a team to treat the child and the parents. His expertise and creative abilities established a coherent, systematic approach to treatment that made therapy more acceptable. He used innovative adaptive equipment to enable his patients to reach their fullest potential and to enjoy a fruitful life. Dr. Phelps is remembered as having contributed precise definitions and classifications for the cerebral palsies. He originated many methods of treatment, refined and improved others, and his standards are the norm from which today's treatment techniques continue to evolve.

APPENDIX I

Outline of 15 treatment modalities described by Dr. Phelps for training therapists (c.f. bibliography and further reading for details).
1. Massage: believed to aid circulation and nutrition of weak muscles, rarely used today with patients having cerebral palsy.
2. Passive motion: done by the therapist to the child for the purpose of developing concepts of correct movements. Timing is important; it is slower with an athetoid child, and performed with a faster rhythm to the spastic child. All movements begin with proximal joints and progress distally for all types of cerebral palsy. Passive motion might also include stretching (very slowly) a spastic muscle, with a gradual increase in range of motion. If a stretch reflex or clonus occurs in the spastic child or involuntary motions are observed in the athetoid child, the exercise is immediately stopped and begun again only after relaxation takes place.
3. Active assistive motion: is done by the therapist with only a little help from the child who is beginning to feel the gravity effects of motion. Again these are immediately discontinued if stretch reflexes or involuntary movements occur.
4. Active motion: is advance voluntary motion when the child has learned control. Range and speed are stressed; with their mastery comes the performance of useful activities.
5. Resisted motion: is movement performed against manual resistance or gravity. They are used generally to increase muscle strength; yet can be carried out to assist the athetoid establish muscle contraction.

6. Conditioned motion: is movement taught the child through rhyme and song by the therapist first doing it passively to the child, then with the child taking an active part through active assistive motion and finally active motion.

7. Automatic motion: is movement used with synergistic group contractions against resistance to achieve a desired motion where voluntary motion is lacking.

8. Combined motion: is movement of two joints taught an action for self help; finger flexion with wrist extension enables one to hold a comb or eat.

9. Rest: is no activity. Some cerebral-palsy children need braces and adaptive furniture to accomplish rest.

10. Relaxation: is taught using Jacobson's progressive method.

11. Motion from a relaxed position: is used mainly with the athetoid child.

12. Balance: is achieving an upright posture in space and follows normal development, sitting, kneeling, standing and on to walking.

13. Reciprocation: is taught when the child is ready to begin walking. Conditioned exercises may be combined here using parallel bars, skis, quad canes *etc*.

14. Reach grasp and release: are taught as a combination of joint motions allowing the child to use his arm in a functional manner. When done seated upright they assist eye-hand co-ordination development.

15. Skills: are taught when joint motions can be performed with rhythmical ease. A skill is any self-help action: self-feeding, dressing, writing, typing, *etc*. (Egel 1948, Jones 1967).

APPENDIX II

Photographs depicting equipment and treatment of the type used by Phelps, furnished through the courtesy of the Illustration Department of the Indiana University School of Medicine. The original pictures were taken between 1936 and 1960 and were released for educational purposes by the Cerebral Palsy Treatment Center, Department of Orthopedics, Indiana University School of Medicine.

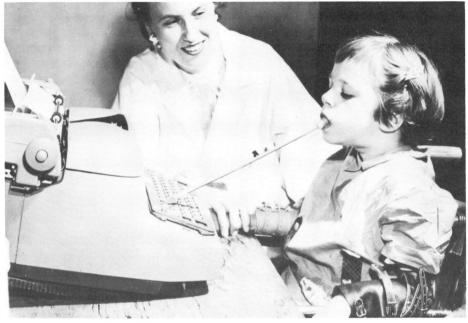

Fig. 1. *Diagnosis:* Flailing athetoid age 7 years.
With Phelps-type forearm stabilizers, she uses her mouth-stick for typing through a keyboard cover. She
   wore full athetoid control braces which guided the development of purposeful tension until age 17.
   Today, in her mid-thirties, she resides in a group home; she uses an adapted wheelchair with ankle
   straps and a free right hand on her communication board/lap-tray. She bears full weight to help
   transfer herself.

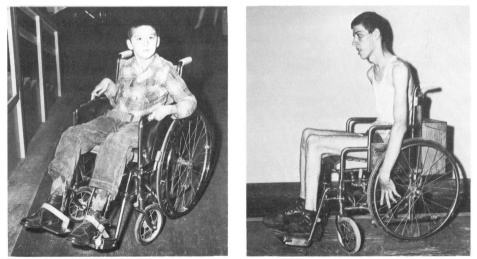

Fig. 2. *Diagnosis:* Quadriplegic rotary athetoid age 11 years.
(a) Wearing Phelps-type waist band, double upright long leg braces with 90° ring locks at hips and 180° at
   both hips and knees. He developed useful tension and control.
(b) Now as an adult of 40 he propels his own chair and is independent in all aspects of self-care. He is
   self-employed, weaving wall-hangings and rugs on consignment on a four or six harness floor loom.

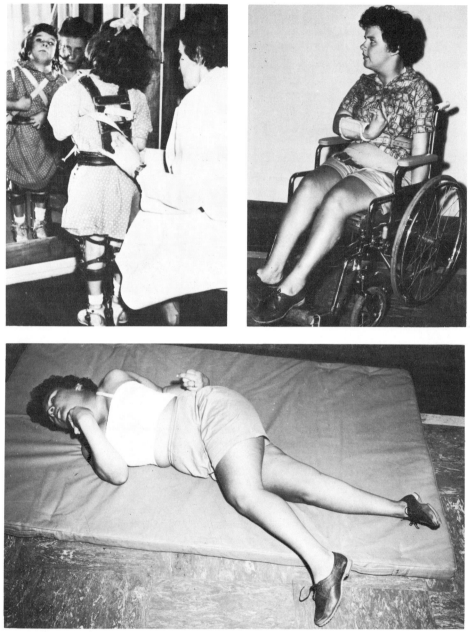

Fig. 3. *Diagnosis:* Flailing athetoid age 4.
(a) Wearing Phelps-type modified back-brace attached to full control double uprights with 90° hip and knee locks for standing.
(b) Developing useful tension and control by age 16, she has progressed to using a standard wheelchair with only arm stabilizers. Today she is in her mid-thirties; she types with a mouth-stick (30 words per minute), and operates a motor-chair with sip and puff and arm cuffs.
(c) Mat position shows tension.

70

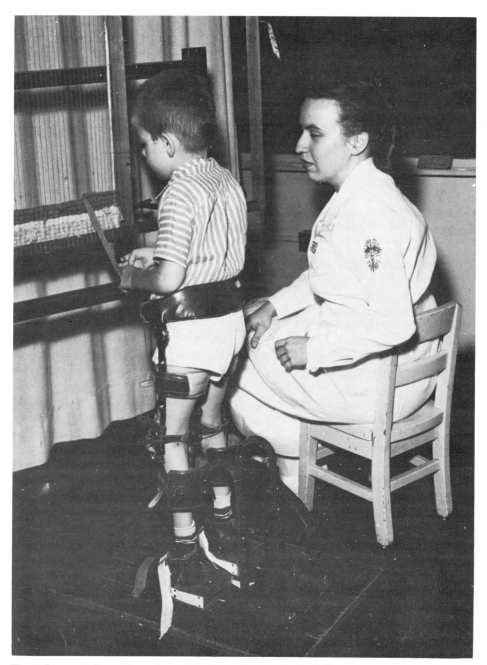

Fig. 4. *Diagnosis:* Boy with atonia, working to develop tension for balance and support. Wearing waist band, Phelps-type braces and standing in a Phelps stabilizer, he learns balance while using his hands on the upright weaving frame. At age 16½ years he had ankle and back fusions. Today at 45 he is a vocational counselor with a Ph.D., he uses two lofstrand canes or a wheelchair. He drives his own hand-controlled automobile.

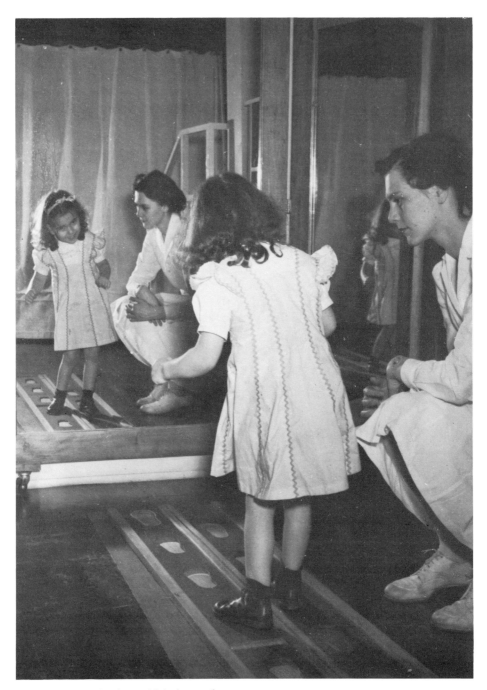

Fig. 5. *Diagnosis:* Ataxic quadriplegic, age 6 years.
Here she is using Phelps-type removable footprints to control stride length and width, as well as to develop reciprocal hip motion and balance. A grandmother at 45, she enjoys life on the farm.

REFERENCES

Brunyate, R. W. (1952) 'Featured occupational therapy departments.' *American Journal of Occupational Therapy*, **6**, 219–227.
—— (1963) 'Occupational therapy for patients with cerebral palsy.' *In:* Willard, H. S., Spackman, C. S. (Eds.) *Occupational Therapy, 3rd Edn.* Philadelphia: Lippincott. pp. 264–307.
Carlson, E. R. (1941) *Born That Way.* New York: Day. pp. 123–124.
Crothers, B., Paine, R. S. (1959) *The Natural History of Cerebral Palsy.* Cambridge, Mass.: Harvard University Press. p. 37.
Denhoff, E., Robinault, I. (1960) 'Clinical descriptions.' *In: Cerebral Palsy and Related Disorders.* New York: McGraw-Hill. pp. 28–39.
Doll, E. E., Walker, M. S. (1951) 'Handedness in cerebral palsied children.' *Journal of Consulting Psychology*, **15**, 9–17.
Egel, P. F. (1948) *Technique of Treatment for the Cerebral Palsy Child.* St. Louis: C. V. Mosby. p. 195.
Fay, T. (1946) 'Problems of rehabilitation in patients with cerebral palsy.' *Delaware Medical Journal*, **18**, 57–60.
—— (1950) 'Cerebral palsy—medical considerations and classification.' *American Journal of Psychiatry*, **107**, 180–183.
—— (1954) 'The use of pathological and unlocking reflexes in the rehabilitation of spastics.' *American Journal of Physical Medicine*, **33**, 347–352.
Gillette, H. E. (1969) *Systems of Therapy in Cerebral Palsy.* Springfield, Ill.: C. C. Thomas.
Hadra, R. (1955, 1966) *In:* Cruickshank, W. M., Raus, G. M. (Eds.) *Cerebral Palsy, its Individual and Community Problems, 1st and 2nd Edns.* Syracuse: Syracuse University Press. p. 440.
Jacobson, E. (1938) *Progressive Relaxation, 2nd Edn.* Chicago: Chicago University Press.
Jones, A. M. (1967) 'The traditional method of treatment for the cerebral palsied child.' *American Journal of Physical Medicine*, **46**, 1024–1031.
Kahmann, W. C. (1938) 'The project for the treatment of cerebral palsy at Riley Hospital.' *Occupational Therapy*, **17**, 89–92.
Lord, E. E. (1937) *Children Handicapped by Cerebral Palsy.* New York: The Commonwealth Fund; London: Oxford University Press. pp. 23–41, 102.
Martin, E. F. (1940) 'Occupational therapy treatment for cerebral palsied at the Children's Rehabilitation Institute.' *Occupational Therapy*, **19**, 331–338.
Miller, A. S., Stewart, M. D., Murphy, M. A., Jantzen, A. C. (1955) 'An evaluation method for cerebral palsy.' *Occupational Therapy*, **9**, 105–112.
National Society for Crippled Children and Adults (1950) *Manual of Cerebral Palsy Equipment.* Chicago: National Society for Crippled Children and Adults.
Phelps, W. M. (1941a) 'Factors influencing the treatment of cerebral palsy.' *Physiotherapy Review*, **21**, 136–138.
—— (1941b) 'The management of the cerebral palsies.' *Journal of the American Medical Association*, **117**, 1612–1625.
—— (1942) 'Recent trends in cerebral palsy.' *Archives of Physical Therapy*, **23**, 332–336.
—— (1947) *The Farthest Corner—an Outline of the Cerebral Palsy Problem, 4th Edn.* New York: National Society for Crippled Children and Adults. pp. 1–23.
—— (1949) 'Description and differentiation of types of cerebral palsy.' *Nervous Child*, **8**, 107–127.
—— (1951) 'Dietary requirements in cerebral palsy.' *Journal of the American Dietetic Association*, **27**, 869–870.
—— (1952) 'Bracing in the cerebral palsies.' *In:* Edwards, J. W. (Ed.) *Orthopedic Appliances Atlas, Vol. I: Braces, Splints, Shoe Alterations.* Ann Arbor, Michigan: Illinois University Press. pp. 521–536.
—— (1957) 'Long-term results of orthopaedic surgery in cerebral palsy.' *Journal of Bone and Joint Surgery*, **39A**, 53–59.
—— Hopkins, T. (1958) *The Cerebral Palsied Child, a Guide for Parents.* New York: Simon & Schuster.
—— (1959) 'Preliminary institutional evaluation of a new drug in cerebral palsy.' *Archives of Pediatrics*, **76**, 243–250.
Price, A. (1954) 'Laterality of upper extremity function in physically handicapped children.' *American Journal of Occupational Therapy*, **8**, 241–259.
Samilson, R. L. (Ed.) (1975) *Orthopedic Aspects of Cerebral Palsy; Clinics in Developmental Medicine Nos. 52/3.* London: S.I.M.P. with Heinemann; Philadelphia: Lippincott. p. 92.
Scherzer, A. L., Tscharnuter, I. (1982) *Early Diagnosis and Therapy in Cerebral Palsy.* New York: Marcel Dekker.

Slominski, A. H. (1950–54) Personal notes from Phelps lecture series given at the Children's Rehabilitation Institute and Columbia University.

—— Hamant, C. (1971) 'Occupational therapy for cerebral palsy'. *In:* Willard, H. S., Spackman, C. S. (Eds.) *Occupational Therapy, 4th Edn.* Philadelphia: Lippincott. pp. 338–372.

Westlake, H. (1951) 'A system for developing speech with the cerebral palsied children.' *Reprinted from: The Crippled Child,* National Society for Crippled Children and Adults, Chicago, Illinois. p. 15.

FURTHER READING

*Especially useful to parents and teachers

*Bleck, E. E., Nagel, D. A. (Eds.) (1975) *Physically Handicapped Children: a Medical Atlas for Teachers.* New York: Grune & Stratton.

*Bratshaw, M. L., Perret, Y. M. (1981) *Children with Handicaps: a Medical Primer.* Baltimore: Brookes.

*Clark, C. A., Chadwick, D. M. (1979) *Clinically Adapted Instruments for the Multiply Handicapped.* Westford, Mass.: Modulations Company.

*Collis, E. (1947) *A Way of Life for the Handicapped Child—a New Approach to Cerebral Palsy.* London: Faber & Faber.

*Cooper, J. M., Morehouse, L. E. (Eds.) (1953) *Assisting the Cerebral Palsied Child—Lifting and Carrying; I: In the House; II: Outside the House.* New York: United Cerebral Palsy Association.

*Copeland, K. (Ed.) (1974) *Aids for the Severely Handicapped.* London: Sector; New York: Grune and Stratton.

Crothers, B. (1923) 'Changes of pressure inside the fetal craniovertebral cavity.' *Journal of Surgery, Gynecology and Obstetrics,* **37,** 790.

Fischel, M. K. (1934) *The Spastic Child.* St Louis: C. V. Mosby.

*Fraser, B. A., Hensinger, R. N. (1983) *Managing Physical Handicaps—a Practical Guide for Parents, Care Providers, and Educators.* Baltimor: Brooks.

Girard, P. M. (1937) *The Home Treatment of Spastic Paralysis.* Philadelphia: Lippincott.

*Goldsmith, S. (1976) *Designing for the Disabled, 3rd Edn.* London: R.I.B.A.

Hadra, R. (1950) 'Developmental factors in the cerebral palsied child.' *The Crippled Child,* **18,** 22–24.

*Hale, G. (Ed.) (1979) *The New Source Book for the Disabled in Britain.* London: Imprint Books. (Bantam edition—July 1981.)

*Kernaleguen, A. (1978) *Clothing Designs for the Handicapped.* Edmonton, Alberta: University of Alberta Press.

*Lowman, E. W., Klinger, J. L. (1969) *Aids to Independent Living—Self-help for the Handicapped.* New York: McGraw-Hill.

*Marks, N. C. (1974) *Cerebral Palsied and Learning Disabled Children—a Handbook/Guide to Treatment, Rehabilitation and Education.* Springfield, Ill.: C. C. Thomas.

Osler, W. (1889) *The Cerebral Palsies of Children. A Clinical Study from the Infirmary for Nervous Diseases.* Philadelphia: Blakiston.

Payton, O. D., Hirt, S., Newton, R. A. (1977) *Scientific Bases for Neurophysiologic Approaches to Therapeutic Excercise—an Anthology.* Philadelphia: F. A. Davis.

Phelps, W. M. (1945) 'The cerebral palsies.' *In:* Mitchell-Nelson, *Textbook of Pediatrics, 4th edn.* Philadelphia: W. B. Saunders. pp. 111–116.

—— (1946) 'Recent significant trends in the care of cerebral palsy.' *Journal of the Southern Medical Association,* **39,** 132-138.

—— (1947) 'Cerebral palsy.' *In:* Whipple, A. O. (Ed.) *Nelson New Loose-Leaf Surgery.* New York: Thomas Nelson. p. 180.

—— (1952) 'General management of the cerebral palsy problem.' *Virginia Medical Monthly,* **79,** 65–69.

—— (1952) 'Braces, upper and lower extremities.' *American Academy of Orthopedic Surgeons, Instructional Course Lectures,* Vols. 9 and 10.

Rogers, G. G., Thomas, L. C. (1935) *New Pathways for Children with Cerebral Palsy.* New York: Macmillan.

Sherrington, C. S. (1907) 'On reciprocal innervation of antagonistic muscles.' *Proceedings of the Royal Society, London,* **79,** 337–349.

—— (1913) 'Reflex inhibitions as a factor in the co-ordination of movements and posture.' *Quarterly Journal of Experimental Physiology,* **6,** 251–253.

—— (1947) *The Integrative Action of the Nervous System, 2nd Edn.* New Haven, Conn: Yale University Press. p. 209.

6

THE BASIC ELEMENTS OF TREATMENT ACCORDING TO VOJTA

Vaclav Vojta

Introduction

Reflex locomotion as a working hypothesis

The traditional way of considering reflex locomotion needs to be reconsidered in the light of recent clinical experience. Locomotion always consists of the following distinct but inseparable elements: (i) automatic control of the body position as a whole; (ii) the uprighting mechanisms necessary for the type of locomotion; (iii) the phasic movements of the particular type of locomotion, which are seen mainly as stepping movements. The term 'reflex locomotion' implies that the total movement pattern does not appear spontaneously but only by stimulation from the periphery, *i.e.* the stimulation of body parts. However the provoked local pattern involves the whole body, including all the extremities. The term also implies that there are several such automatic global patterns, each with its own separate characteristics.

We have studied these movement patterns closely for many years among children with cerebral palsy, from preschool age up to 15 years (Vojta 1962, 1964, 1965) and have noted that some of the postures which can be observed spontaneously or provoked with older cerebral-palsied children are already apparent in abnormal infants and even abnormal newborns (Vojta 1968, 1969*b*, 1970, 1981). This leads us to consider that the postural control mechanisms within the central nervous system of a cerebral-palsied *child* have something in common with those of the central nervous system of a pathological *newborn* (Vojta 1981). The spontaneous movements of a normal newborn therefore might be of decisive importance in understanding the dynamics of a cerebral paretic disturbance. Furthermore, an understanding of pathological movement might in turn contribute to the understanding of normal motor development.

Rationale

The earliest stages of movement development

Daily clinical experience shows that movements which can be provoked and observed (segment by segment and muscle by muscle) in cerebral-palsied children can be seen instantly in healthy newborns. From this it might be concluded that the muscle work found with such abundance in the newborn, and provoked by reflexes from a cerebral-palsied child, have a common neurogenic pattern in the sub-cortex, not in the motor cortex (Vojta *et al.* 1967, Vojta 1969*a*). Thus among a cerebral-palsied patient's motor abilities there might be movement patterns from his newborn period which can be provoked and activated. If these movement patterns in the newborn are global, and if they contain components of locomotion,

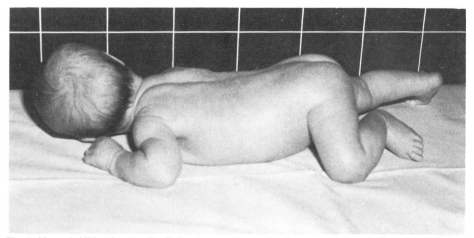

Fig. 1. Normal child at four weeks. Extension movement of left arm, carried out by long head of triceps muscle, occurs in frontal plane of body.

then even a newborn must have reached a certain maturity of postural ontogenesis. Consequently, the persistence in cerebral-palsied patients of the movement patterns of a disturbed newborn is the outcome of nothing other than the blocking of postural ontogenesis during the earliest period of human motor development (Vojta 1981).

Developmental kinesiology and the earliest acquisition of control of uprighting and equilibrium
A further decisive concept was arrived at from the working hypothesis of reflex locomotion; each method of locomotion involves its own regular reciprocal change of limb position and of the body's centre of gravity. This flowing, supple change of the centre of gravity—called 'equilibrium'—requires that the extremities have fixed points external to the body axis. If cerebral-palsied children are typified by a deficiency of equilibrium, and if inherent global patterns with components of locomotion can be provoked in normal newborns (Vojta 1966, 1968, 1970), it is conceivable that one might influence a mechanism which involves the control not only of the body position but also of the centre of gravity, *i.e.* the equilibrium (Vojta 1966). From this can be deduced a further concept: that the equilibrium reactions are present in normal development (Vojta 1981), even in its earliest stages (Vojta 1962, 1964). This working hypothesis of the inherent locomotion pattern gave an insight into the earliest acquisition of the uprighting mechanism and the control of equilibrium.

Differentiation of muscle functions
Shifting the centre of gravity by reflex locomotion patterns is possible only if a point of support is created on the body or on the extremities. For example, in reflex creeping (Fig. 1) the elbow can be this *punctum fixum*. However, for the newborn

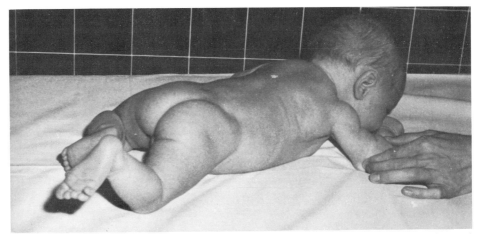

Fig. 2. Normal child at four weeks. In the scheme of reflex creeping, using the medial humeral epicondylar zone, all three parts of triceps muscle are contracted, with flexed elbow. Note that head rotates to left, trunk becomes supported on elbow, and trunk (thorax) rotates to left. The centre of gravity is shifted laterally to right side.

and during the first four to six weeks of life, the spontaneous extension movement of the arm is pointed backward at the shoulder joint.

In the reflex creeping pattern the muscle triceps brachii, for example, contracts; but because of the elbow's support the action of this muscle has changed fundamentally from that of the spontaneous contraction seen in Figure 1. As a muscle always contracts towards the *punctum fixum*, in the reflex creeping pattern the triceps brachii is contracted towards the elbow (Fig. 2). This is a completely different muscle action from that of a normal newborn or infant, as well as some children with cerebral palsy; when they move their arms backwards spontaneously in prone (Fig. 1) they extend their arms with the long head of triceps brachii and the movement occurs in the frontal plane. The action is similar in supine.

In the reflex creeping pattern, however, the contraction and the provocable movement is almost in the sagittal plane of the body. With the newborn, by fixing the elbow (Fig. 3e) the movement occurs at the shoulder joints, but now it is the body which is moving towards the arm. The body is lifted over the lever of the upper arm and pulled forward in a cranial and lateral direction; this can be considered as an uprighting movement.

What is even more important is that with this process there is a certain differentiation of muscle function which would never occur spontaneously in a cerebral-palsied child. With the help of the reflex locomotion pattern it is possible to isolate the function of each skeletal muscle of a cerebral-palsied child, not only in the area of the shoulder joints but throughout the extremities.

Treatment
Activation of the central nervous system
By applying these patterns of reflex locomotion to isolate different muscle

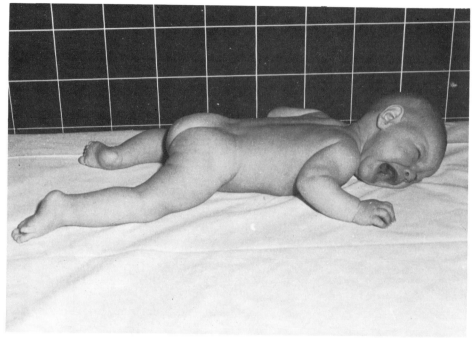

Fig. 3a. Child of nine months with spastic diplegia.

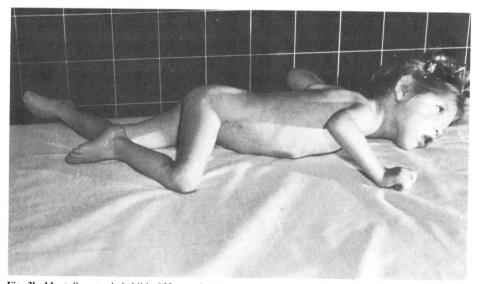

Fig. 3b. Mentally retarded child of 32 months with spastic tetraplegia. Extension of arm is carried out in frontal plane of body—just as by child in first weeks of life. This child has limited head movement and here uses lateral elevation of head to orient eyes. Primitive asymmetrical rotation of head remains unchanged. Her needs for visual orientation and communication with her surroundings forces her to practise and perfect this inadequate and primitive posture.

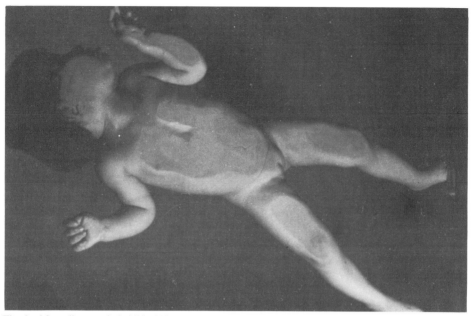

Fig. 3c. Mentally retarded child of 20 months with spastic diplegia, seen from below lying on glass plate, showing unsupported primitive pattern of an arm, with retraction, *i.e.* extension, of the arm at the shoulder joint.

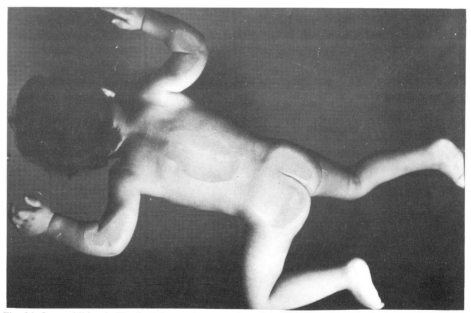

Fig. 3d. Same child as in Fig. 3c, lying supine on a glass plate. Primitive pattern of arms, ventral flexion of pelvis, reclination of head and the kyphosis of trunk are evident by seeing the child from below.

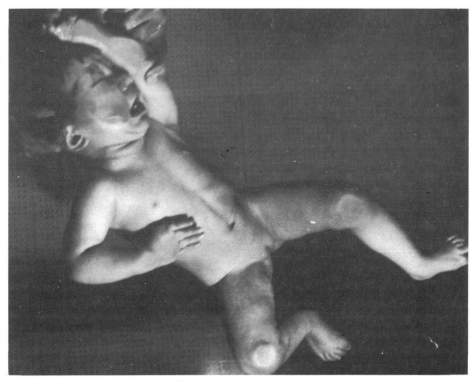

Fig. 3e. Same child as in Figs. 3c and d, using medial humeral epincondylar trigger zone. By resisting reflex rotation of head to left, the trunk is lifted and rotated to left, with support on right elbow. Pelvis is flexed dorsally by massive contraction of the ventral layer of muscles. Note expansion of thorax (ideal configuration of body), and in orofacial area shift of mouth to left, *i.e.* in direction of rotary process. Left arm is moving forward, hand is extending at wrist-joint, and fingers are extending. In the right leg there is ideal contraction of the whole adductor group—in synergistic function with flexion of leg, including hip joint.
Note: Contact area of cheek is smaller than in Fig. 3c, although movement of head is resisted (see therapist's hand).

functions in children with cerebral palsy, we can activate: (i) postural ontogenesis, (ii) the uprighting mechanism and (iii) the equilibrium reaction, on the assumption that there are neuronal reserves in the central nervous system. Using the activatory system of reflex locomotion, the child can develop its postural and locomotion ontogenesis.

Shifting possibilities in the neuronal structure of the global pattern
The co-ordination complexes of reflex locomotion are global patterns, which can be activated by different reflexogenic zones. For instance when activating a global pattern it is possible, by concentrating on any one component of the complex (*e.g.* the uprighting component) to activate the other two, the phasic and postural components. The ability to activate the same global movement outcome from different points means that with a combination of these zones the reaction—the

movement desired—can be obtained quicker and more precisely.

Early in the development of this treatment method we noted the following:
(1) If one zone gave only little or no response, another point of stimulation was taken and the reaction appeared: if these two zones were combined (the active and the inactive zone simultaneously) the activation increased in its intensity.
(2) The inactive zone *suddenly* became active, especially in young infants.

We explained these observations by the hypothesis that the central co-ordination of the whole neuronal structure of the pattern is changed. Some connections were being activated which had previously been inactive and/or impermeable; a potential blockade had been overcome. In other words it is possible (i) to activate the central nervous system, (ii) to awaken it from a disturbed situation, and (iii) to guide it towards normal development.

Such a statement might sound bold had it not been arrived at through an empirical approach to our regular clinical practice. Perhaps a better explanation for our observations will be found, but for the time being it is the best we have come across.

Different ways of obtaining the same pattern
By combining zones it is possible to increase the excitation of the central nervous system by spatial summation. There are different points of excitation in the patterns of reflex creeping and reflex turning. In the first pattern there are nine such points or areas of excitation (or as we say 'trigger zones'). In the other pattern there are also nine trigger zones if one includes the side-lying position. These nine trigger zones can be used either alone or in combination, as well as in different sequences, so there are thousands of possibilities of activating the central nervous system. If it is possible to activate the same global pattern—by a modest estimation—in 50,000 different ways to create it in its globality, then the same pattern is activated in its globality. However, both its temporal storage in the central nervous system and the method of activation of its individual parts are stored in a separate manner for each different possibility.

Our patterns are reciprocal ones: the final position of the preceding cycle is the starting position of the reverse cycle (Fig. 4). Imprinting in the central nervous system is reflected in both hemispheres of the cerebrum, which of course are interconnected. It appears that the intensity of the imprinting of these reciprocal patterns is not increased arithmetically (*i.e.* doubled), but rather geometrically.

The outcome of activation of an inherent pattern by temporal summation
The intensity of the provoked movement can be increased by being resisted. If the resistance is so strong that movement cannot occur, then the previous isotonic muscle contraction becomes an isometric contraction. This does not obstruct activation. On the contrary, it highlights a fact fundamental to reciprocal movements; as long as one remains in the starting position the goal is always 'anticipated'.

We consider that the effect of long-term excitation of isometric contraction in the starting position is a summation of the excitation in the central nervous system;

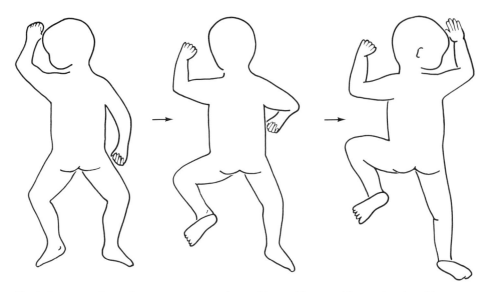

Fig. 4. Sequence of creeping movements: starting position, midway position, and end position.

we are then working with temporal summation. While holding this posture, proprioceptive information is being continuously offered for processing to the central nervous system, reflecting the activity produced in the periphery. When all this proprioceptive information is multiplied by the time factor, the temporal summation in our pattern suddenly becomes an imprinting factor. As the majority of the excitations are proprioceptive and are constant, or only slightly variable, temporal summation becomes the most important factor in the activation of the central nervous system.

Imprinting new muscle patterns in the central nervous system
The image of the normal newborn projected into the disturbed central nervous system
The global patterns of reflex locomotion can be elicited easily from a normal newborn. With the disturbed infant, or one with established cerebral palsy*, the muscle action of the global patterns cannot be provoked so easily or to their full extent. However, provided the therapist knows the exact starting position, she can (through temporal or spatial summation) activate the muscles to contract isometrically because this starting position is part of the pattern of a normal infant. Such activity in the peripheral motor system is a source of new global proprioception which is transmitted to the central nervous system, where it is stored. If the starting position is a physiological one, then the state of the activation

---

**Editor's note:* Dr. Vojta uses the term 'disturbed infant' to describe the cerebral-palsied infant who as yet has had no opportunity to practise and establish pathological movement patterns. 'Established' or 'fixed' cerebral palsy refers to the older child who has established such pathological patterns.

of the muscles, the tension of the tendon, and the proprioception of the joints and articular capsules is transmitted simultaneously and as a whole to the central nervous system.

A competent therapist can produce within the central nervous system the postural experiences of a normal infant (*e.g.* uprighting mechanisms) which otherwise would never occur from the spontaneous movements of a pathological infant or one with cerebral palsy. In this way the initial phase of normal motor ontogenesis is activated. The following phases of ontogenesis develop spontaneously within the central nervous system.

The use of imprinted patterns in spontaneous movement
The global patterns are stored in their individual component parts in the huge treasury of the central nervous system—provided there is sufficient neuronal mass and a certain degree of plasticity in the central nervous system. If these partial patterns are stored individually, it follows that they can be used individually by the central nervous system in spontaneous movement. It would be easy to argue with this concept were it not supported by daily clinical experience and also by the most recent neurophysiological concepts (Evarts and Tanji 1979). If in the reflex creeping pattern, for example, radial fist closure exists as a partial pattern of a global pattern, and if this partial pattern can be stored individually, then with correct motivation a radial hand closure (fist closure) is possible, provided there is the involuntary ability for spontaneous grasping. This too corresponds to clinical experience. When the idea of the global patterning of human motor ontogenesis first emerged, no one was practising grasping with cerebral-palsied children, nor was anyone practising standing and walking exercises or training for sitting or chewing. The children had to discover these functions for themselves from the elements of the reflex locomotion patterns.

Motor activity anticipated in the formation of bipedal locomotion
The global patterns of reflex locomotion exist in their entirety in each healthy newborn; or rather, they can be provoked. It was ascertained that by activating them in a pathological infant or in a child with established cerebral palsy, the initial phase of normal motor ontogenesis was awakened.

It was mentioned earlier that the cerebral-palsied children invent various motor functions spontaneously after being activated with these global patterns, provided sufficient cortex remains intact. This statement needs explanation. Analysis of these global patterns (Vojta 1965, 1966, 1969, 1971, 1981) shows that the elements—the partial patterns— are produced spontaneously during normal motor development in the first year of life. In the reflex creeping pattern, for example, there is an element of the phase of verticality around the pelvic girdle. It is by this means that the entry into the fourth trimenan or the end of the third trimenan is 'anticipated' within the organisation of the newborn infant.

In the reflex creeping pattern, for example, the partial pattern of the foot is kinesiologically the same as the movement of the foot rolling from heel to toe in bipedal locomotion. Consequently we speak of 'anticipation' of the partial pattern of bipedal locomotion extending to the end of the first year of life and into the fifth trimenan.

However, an exact knowledge of the global pattern is of the utmost importance. A child (even with an already developed cerebral palsy) who has achieved the ability to stand and to skip on one leg during therapy has already escaped the level of serious motor dysfunction, by which I mean he has escaped cerebral palsy; he has achieved the motoric differentiation of the legs. Furthermore, if a child, through therapy, has achieved the skill of correct radial gripping, this child also is out of the realms of grave motor disorder of central origin—that is, cerebral palsy. This is because it is our consistent experience that he can use the upper extremities as fully developed catching tools and also has the ability to recognise objects stereognostically.

I have referred above only to the most obvious characteristics of gross motor development, the individual elements of which can be activated by the co-ordination complexes of reflex locomotion. It must not be forgotten, however, that cerebral palsy is a disturbance of gross motor *development*. If the precursors of motor ontogenesis already exist within the central nervous system, then it is the physiotherapist's task to activate the system to combine these elements, using spatial and temporal summation.

Teaching parents to treat their child
The therapist requires a full knowledge of the patterns of reflex locomotion, and of their selection and use in treatment; however, once the treatment for a particular child has been selected, the technique itself is surprisingly easy to learn. For this reason the frequency of instruction by the therapist needs to be no more than twice or at the most four times a month for infants, and only once every four to six weeks for older children. However, the instruction must be precise and it is important that sufficient time is allocated at each session so that parents can learn the exercises faultlessly. Parents can be exceedingly effective therapists using this treatment, so it is surprisingly economical and efficient.

Effects of the therapy
Naturally there is a difference between the results of treatment for those with fixed and those with impending cerebral palsy. Children with fixed cerebral palsies show objective improvement only after months of treatment, while infants can show improvement within a few weeks.

As a rule, if no significant improvement can be seen after treating a child persistently for a year, it is assumed that the limits of treatment have been reached. To apply this statement clinically, of course the physician has to have complete confidence in his therapists, and so must demand from them a high level of professional knowledge and competence.

Summary
The application of patterns of reflex locomotion can be seen as a general principle of treatment for motor dysfunction. This treatment was first used for fixed cerebral

palsies, then for pathological newborns and infants. This experience led to certain developmental kinesiological conclusions and provided further insight into human motor ontogenesis. This chapter has referred almost exclusively to the treatment of cerebral palsy, but this method also has increased our understanding of all areas of pathological movement development.

REFERENCES

Evarts, E. V., Tanji, H. (1979) 'Brain mechanisms of movement.' *Scientific American*, **241** (3), 146–156.
Vojta, V. (1962) 'Ontogeny of infantile spasticity.' *(Czech.) Paper presented to the Neurologic Society of ČSSR, Prague.*
—— (1965) 'Reflex loosening of spastic hypertonia.' *(Czech.) Ceskoslovenska Neurologie*, **27**, 229.
—— (1965) 'Rehabilitation in infantile spasticity.' *(German.) Beitrage für Orthopädie und Traumatologie*, **12**, 557–562.
—— (1966) 'Reflex creeping in the rehabilitation of motor disturbance in childhood.' *(Czech.) Ceskoslovenska Neurologie*, **29**, 234–239.
—— (1968) 'Reflex creeping and its importance in early physiotherapy.' *(German.) Zeitschrift für Kinderheilkunde*, **104**, 319–330.
—— (1969a) 'A new position reaction in the early diagnosis of cerebral palsy in the newborn or very young baby.' *(German.) Zeitschrift für Orthopädie*, **107**, 1–11.
—— (1969b) 'Creeping as a component part of rehabilitation therapy of motor disturbance in children.' *In: The Use of Reflex Mechanisms in Re-education of Mobility.* Prague: Balnea. p. 286.
—— (1970) 'Reflex turning as the facilitatory system in human locomotion.' *(German.) Zeitschrift für Orthopädie*, **108**, 446–452.
—— (1981) *Die zerebralen Bewegungsstörungen im Säuglingsalter: Frühdiagnose und Frühtherapie, 3rd Edn.* Stuttgart: Enke.
—— Vele, F., Ackermannová, B. (1967) 'EMG evaluation of special treatment technique used in children with signs of spasticity in cerebral palsy.' *Paper presented at the 2nd International Symposium of Cerebral Palsy, Prague.*

7

SENSORY INTEGRATIVE THERAPY FOR THE CEREBRAL-PALSIED CHILD

Rosemary White

Aims

Sensory integration refers to the ability to organize sensory input for use. The theory evolved from the study of perceptual disorders among children with a diagnosis of cerebral palsy, the area originally studied being visual perception. This work, conducted during the 1950s, was concerned primarily with the study of functional difficulties resulting from poor perception of visual figure-ground, visual space and form in space. It resulted in the realization that functional problems associated with visual perception disorders were only one aspect of a more central underlying neurological dysfunction.

Subsequent research, on which sensory integrative theory is based, was conducted with learning-disabled children, who present with specific perceptual disorders affecting their functional abilities. Furthermore, such children generally do not have other obvious signs of neurological dysfunction likely to affect the results of studies. The emphasis of this research was the study of the phylogenically older sensory systems which provide us with fundamental information about ourselves and our environment; in particular, the proprioceptive, tactile and vestibular systems.

The proprioceptive system provides information about muscles and joints, accurately locating the position of one part of the body in relation to others, and in relation to gravity. The tactile system provides information about the contact of the skin with the external environment. These two systems together allow us to perceive our movements and the environment with which we are constantly interacting. The vestibular system, the most recent to be studied, is considered to be an essential integrating system. It provides sensory information about movement of the head and body in space, and the direction of that movement in all planes. As this information is perceived, appropriate postural responses are made, including those of the trunk and limbs as well as the eyes.

The integration of sensation occurs within the brainstem, from where information descends and ascends. The descending information is both facilitatory and inhibitory, affecting responses in the skeletal musculature and in the receptors of the skin. The ascending information allows us to develop a concept by integrating the diffuse sensory information to make a meaningful whole. This information reaches all levels of the central nervous system, and permits continual adjustment of our response to, and perception of, the environment.

Sensory integrative dysfunction refers to an inability to use sensation

86

effectively to make an appropriate response. Dysfunction may involve one or more sensory systems and affect responses at a postural or a conceptual level, thus affecting functional ability during any tasks which depend on information involving the disordered sensory system.

The central principle in sensory integrative therapy is providing planned and controlled sensory input with usually—but not invariably—the eliciting of a related adaptive response in order to enhance the organization of brain mechanisms. The plan includes utilization of neurophysiological mechanisms in a manner that reflects some aspect of the developmental sequence. The objective is progressive organization of the brain in a method as similar to the normal developmental process as is possible (Ayres 1972, p. 114).

Sensory integrative processes have a developmental sequence which courses with the motor development and which generally is not considered in exercise. Therapy does not ask the child for a complicated motor plan or execution unless simpler and ontogenetically earlier ones have been mastered as well as possible. Treatment seeks responses that reflect better sensory integration and more normal patterns of sensory input as opposed to improved motor skill for the sake of skill itself. The motor response carries a meaning in that it provokes sensory input, helps organize it, and provides an overt manifestation of neural integration (Ayres 1972, p. 114–115).

Anticipated changes that may occur as a result of sensory integrative therapy may influence postural responses, environmental awareness or the ability to motor plan an action (see p. 91) and these changes may be seen both during and outside therapy. Such improvements assist the child in developing a more efficient foundation for functional activity, and so better cognitive development. However, improvement in cognitive development occurs only when the presenting delay is the result of poor sensory processing.

Rationale
To appreciate fully the significance of the use of sensory integrative therapy in the treatment of the cerebral-palsied child, the rôle of the sensory systems in normal development must be considered. This chapter emphasises their rôle in motor development, as it is in this area that the cerebral-palsied child experiences greatest difficulty.

As the brain evolved, adding more complex structures to deal with the environment more effectively, a change in the potential for motor output also occurred. The brainstem is primarily concerned with total massive patterning involving overt responses of the entire body, determined by a relatively simple integration [i.e. primitive reflexes and righting reactions]. The advent of the cerebral hemispheres enabled more discrete, individualistic motor patterns based on more precise interpretation of sensory information [i.e. equilibrium reactions] (Ayres 1972, p. 11–12).

Primitive reflexes

At birth the infant has poorly controlled movements which reflect the level of maturation of the central nervous system. Motor behavior is dominated by primitive reflexes, which assist the child's early survival and provide the foundation for motor and cognitive development.

The primitive (brainstem) reflexes are postural and behavioral responses to sensory stimuli. There are many primitive reflexes, but those most relevant to this chapter are rooting, sucking, Moro, asymmetrical tonic neck and tonic labyrinthine (Prechtl and Beintema 1968). These reflexes emerge in the infant in response to tactile, proprioceptive and/or vestibular stimulation, and are most clearly seen during the first five months of life. After that time, although they remain an essential part of the quality of movement, they are integrated and generally are more difficult to elicit. Integration of the infant's primitive reflexes indicates an increased ability to discriminate sensory information, to inhibit responses to some stimuli and to facilitate more selective responses to others. It is at this stage that righting reactions begin to develop.

Righting reactions

Righting reactions serve the function of maintaining normal alignment of the body parts to one another, and the normal orientation of the head within space. These brainstem reactions emerge initially in the prone and supine positions and are fully developed in these positions by the time the infant is six months old. They continue to develop in the posturally more demanding positions, through to standing, until the child is about five years old. The sensory impulses which elicit these responses originate in the otolithic organs of the vestibular system, the tactile receptors in the trunk and the proprioceptors in the neck, as well as from visual cues (Rushworth 1971). The righting reactions include neck righting, head righting on the body and body righting on the head, body righting on the body and optical righting. They describe the early development of motor control in a cephalocaudal pattern, with development of segmentation in the body occurring in vertical, lateral and rotational planes. The development of these reactions indicates maturation of the infant's response to sensory stimuli: he changes from primitive reflex reactions to more discriminative responses as one body part posturally adapts to movement of another body part or to the pull of gravity.

As the righting reactions develop they enable the infant to roll over, move to sitting, four-point kneeling, half-kneeling and standing, and to ambulate with rotation around the body axis and with increasing extension against gravity. Once the child has developed his righting reactions in a particular posture he begins to develop his equilibrium reactions.

Equilibrium reactions

Equilibrium reactions are higher-level cortical reactions which require sensory information to be processed at all levels of the central nervous system. They maintain or regain balance once the center of gravity has been displaced. They occur in the presence of normal muscle tone, and require total integration of responses from the body parts. An equilibrium reaction is made up of all the righting reactions working together, and so is an organized postural response to multisensory information. They begin to develop at around six months of age in prone and supine, and are well developed in all positions by the time the child is five years old.

There are two types of equilibrium reactions: (i) when the individual moves on a stable surface, *e.g.* when crawling, walking or climbing stairs and (ii) when the individual is stable but the supporting surface, such as a car or a boat, is moving. An equilibrium reaction is a smooth, co-ordinated response to changing sensory stimulation and is controlled with a balance between flexor and extensor muscle groups. If when balance is disturbed the sensory stimulation is too overwhelming (*i.e.* movement is too sudden, or push too strong), the individual will lose equilibrium and revert to more primitive righting reactions, or even primitive reflex responses for protection.

To visualize clearly the components that contribute to a pattern of controlled movement, one can envisage a movie of someone getting up from a chair. The entire movie is a movement pattern, and each frame is an equilibrium reaction, made up of all of the righting reactions working together. Righting reactions are integrated primitive reflexes, which are organized postural responses to changes in sensory stimuli.

> Gravity, sounds, sights, tactile stimuli, and those arising from the muscles and related structures impose themselves upon the child, making demands upon him that help determine the nature of growth of the nervous system. The child's innate drives and neural capacity lead him to an abundance of responses, many of them involving maximal effort, that enable him to master those demands and result in experiences that foster his development . . . It is the organizing of successful or adaptive responses to environmental demands that has pushed the progress of evolution of the brain to the point where it is now. (Ayres 1972, p. 11).

The infant develops increased ability to respond more discriminantly to sensory stimuli as his brain matures; he achieves this by his interaction with the environment and the interaction of the environment with him. The mother's interaction with her infant provides constant stimulation to the tactile, proprioceptive and vestibular systems, as well to the more obvious visual, auditory and olfactory systems. The mother rocks, holds, caresses and croons to her infant. The maturation of the central nervous system from the primitive state to the more mature state is a process of inhibition and integration. Abuladze (1968) stated that: 'There are no special inhibitory formations in the central nervous system but the process of inhibition that occurs within it is always associated with the process of stimulation'. Korner and Grobstein (1966) investigated the effects of soothing on visual alertness in infants and concluded that picking up and putting the crying newborn to the shoulder, actions which stimulate the vestibular apparatus, induced a state of visual alertness. This input, vestibular and tactile (from the physical contact) triggered a neurophysiological mechanism which lowered the infant's state of arousal from one of crying to that of alert inactivity.

The process of providing sensory stimulation in an attempt to alter the state of the infant's behavior can be seen very clearly in his everyday handling. As he becomes distressed, the mother attempts to calm him: she rocks her child gently, moving him rhythmically back and forth, providing vestibular stimulation. The movement may be slow or rapid; she may swing the infant up and down in wide arcs or bounce him on her lap in her attempt to calm him. She holds the infant firmly, supporting the head and trunk, providing tactile and proprioceptive stimulation to these central areas of the body. Her aim is to assist him to calm himself, that is to facilitate a more organized state of control. The type of stimulation she provides depends on the child's response and she adjusts her input according to that response. When the infant is calm and alert the mother again adapts her handling: her movements may then become more stimulating or more challenging to his postural responses. She may gradually move her hands so that they provide less support and the infant has to work more independently to maintain postural control. If the infant is able to process the sensory stimulation he adjusts his posture appropriately, remains calm and alert and often shows enjoyment with the stimulation. However, if the demands are too great he loses postural and often emotional control. In response the mother adapts her handling, and provides the stimulation which she has discovered to have a more inhibitory effect on her infant's central nervous system.

The interaction between sensory stimulation and the infant's maturing behavioral response is constant throughout development, and is reflected in motor development by the integration of primitive reflexes and the emergence of righting and equilibrium reactions. These reactions are merely a classification for the organization of postural responses to change in sensory stimulation. Primitive reflexes are the most immature responses; as maturation occurs the infant begins to inhibit these reflexes and to develop righting reactions, which are more discriminative responses to changing sensory stimulation. As further maturation of the central nervous system occurs, the infant develops equilibrium reactions which are the most discriminative responses to changing stimulation. This progression is part of a developmental continuum, and responses can spiral upward or downward depending on the ability to integrate sensory stimuli in a given situation. When stimuli are integrated the response will be the most mature, but if the stimulus is too excitatory the infant reverts to a more primitive response.

The development of postural control enables the infant to explore and interact with objects within the environment. He takes great pleasure in moving and in challenging his ability to control that movement. As he interacts with an object he feels it, exploring its many facets with his fingers and mouth. He may play in this manner for hours on end, constantly discovering new information about the object. He will then move the object, or himself in relation to the object, providing more varied sensory stimulation to the vestibular, proprioceptive and tactile systems. Following this extensive sensory exploration, the infant begins to perceive visual information in a more complex manner: he can now associate color and shape with how an object feels, how it moves, how heavy it is and how it relates to himself and to other objects within the environment, so developing a concept of the object. Subsequently the child can draw on previous experience and eventually recognize an object by vision alone, associating similar shapes and objects. The sight of such objects will evoke concepts of touch, weight and function associated with the earlier sensory exploration of the object. As the infant matures and childhood experiences broaden, he develops more abstract concepts. This early vestibular, proprioceptive and tactile play enables the child to develop the form and space perception that is the foundation for complex manipulative skills and for later abstract concepts, such as letter and number recognition.

An important result of the sensory integrative process is the ability to motor plan: 'That is the ability of the brain to conceive of, organize, and carry out a sequence of unfamiliar actions' (Ayres 1979). As the infant moves parts of his body in relation to each other and gravity, as well touching himself from head to toe, he begins to develop a body scheme, an internal map of himself. This map becomes more detailed as the infant develops the ability to discriminate sensory information: he then begins to perceive where his body and the external environment begin and end. This perception is a function of the tactile and proprioceptive systems, and is essential if the child is to be able to develop skilled movement. As the infant moves his body during the early months of life and during initial play with toys, his movements reflect the patterns of his primitive reflexes. Once he has integrated all the sensory information from an interaction—that is, explored the tactile, proprioceptive, vestibular, visual, auditory and olfactory sensations— he can develop a concept of that action or object. He is then ready to plan his motor reactions in relation to the object. The infant may hold a rattle, look at it and hear its sounds, but he will not shake it purposefully to make sounds or watch the parts move until he has been able to integrate all those senses into a meaningful concept. This process continues throughout development and is a necessary component of all functional activity. 'The young child motor plans putting on clothes, writing the alphabet, and speaking in complete sentences. Learning to use a new tool requires motor planning. At that time he pays attention to every movement and every sense related to the task, and cannot pay attention to anything else. Attention enables the brain to plan the kind of messages to send to the muscles and the sequence in which to send them' (Ayres 1979). Once the skill has been mastered the actions become automatic and no longer require planning.

An example of early motor planning is seen when the infant learns 'pat-a-cake'. The infant begins to engage the hands in midline at around six to eight weeks: he will then grasp objects and handle them in the midline, and bring them to his mouth. He follows this sequence of play when he develops postural control in sitting. During this time the mother may sing songs to the infant and incorporate hand actions, but the infant is unable to initiate those actions or complete the sequence independently. At around 36 weeks, however, as he begins to be able to clap his hands purposefully, he is able to motor plan the task. The mother will then accompany the infant's hand-clapping with 'pat-a-cake', and the infant will associate the skilled motor act that he has executed independently with the song.

When he is able to respond to the auditory cue of the song with the appropriate motor act, the process has become automatic.

The child's independence in dressing relies on the ability to motor plan. He not only requires the motor skills of being able to flex and extend his limbs; he must also be able to perceive the shape of the clothing and where to place his limbs in relation to the parts of the clothing. It is a complex motor skill which only becomes automatic for the child after about three years of constant daily experience.

Sensory integration is a complex process which influences all aspects of development. Dysfunction in the ability to process sensory information may affect the function of other brain structures. When a child presents with cerebral palsy, one must consider all levels of neurological function during evaluation. Although the major area of dysfunction may involve the motor cortex, there may be specific or associated dysfunction within the brainstem. Recognition of this area of dysfunction will enable the parent, doctor and therapist to treat the child in a more comprehensive manner and help the child to achieve a higher level of function.

Treatment

The child with cerebral palsy may have sensory integrative dysfunction as a result of neurological dysfunction within the brainstem or limited sensory experience from lack of normal motor control. Sensory integrative dysfunction can lead to inadequate inhibition of primitive reflexes, and therefore can delay motor development. It can also affect the child's ability to interpret sensations and use them to form meaningful concepts, which are necessary for learning and motor planning. This includes simple tasks as well as the more complex learning associated with formal education.

When evaluating the cerebral-palsied child, the therapist observes the child's spontaneous movements to determine how efficiently he has integrated his primitive reflexes and developed his righting and equilibrium reactions. The level of maturation of motor development is an indicator of central nervous system function. It describes how well the child is able to discriminate sensory information; the more complex his responses, the more efficiently he is able to discriminate multisensory information. The therapist then observes the child's response to sensory stimuli by moving him from one position to another, or moving him on a surface such as a ball. Postural and behavioral responses are noted in response to this changing vestibular, proprioceptive and tactile stimulation. Formal testing with the Southern California Sensory Integration Tests and the Southern California Postrotatory Nystagmus Test may be appropriate, but these are standardized tests which require completion of all test items without undue interference from abnormal motor activity. This is seldom the case for the cerebral-palsied child, so clinical observations and evaluation from parental interview usually have to suffice.

The environment for sensory integrative therapy looks much the same as a play-area in a park, and is equally appealing to the child. Equipment is designed to provide vestibular stimulation, so there are swings, hammocks and balls to lie or sit or stand on. There is also equipment to provide proprioceptive stimulation. Many of the swings are springy, to provide the same sort of muscle and joint stimulation that the child provides himself with as he rocks back and forth, up and down or side to side. There is also equipment to provide tactile stimulation, and many of the swings are covered with materials of various textures. There may also be areas in which the child can immerse himself uninhibitedly in an environment which will give tactile stimulation to his entire body, such as a young child seeks out for himself in sand or water. Although the therapeutic environment looks like any other play-area, it has been designed to meet the needs of children having difficulty in responding to sensation appropriately. The rôle of the therapist is to manipulate the environment so that the child can achieve his highest level of response, and so promote the development of more mature neural function. The therapist therefore must have a good knowledge of the development of sensory processing, and of how it affects adaptive responses, both posturally and behaviorally.

The sensory integrative therapist's rôle with the cerebral-palsied child is more specialized than that with the child presenting only with a specific dysfunction of sensory integration. It is my opinion that children with cerebral-palsy need correct handling during sensory integrative therapy, and the combination of 'neuro-developmental' (Bobath) handling and sensory integrative therapy is a most effective treatment. The child should be handled smoothly, around 'key points of control'. Movement may be fast or slow, but always rhythmical and sensitive to the child's postural and behavioral responses. In many ways this framework is similar to the maternal handling described earlier in this chapter. As the child responds more appropriately to the sensory input, the therapist adapts her control, perhaps moving her hands distally and allowing the child to control himself proximally. If the child then loses postural control (because the sensory stimulation is too overwhelming) the therapist reverts to more proximal control, and changes the sensory stimulation to inhibit the child's central nervous system.

Example

Andy is a five-year-old boy with quadriplegic cerebral palsy, having greater dysfunction on the right side of the body. He is able to roll over, crawl and come to sitting independently, rotating to the right side. He can sit independently for a few moments. He has retained the tonic labyrinthine, asymmetrical tonic neck and Moro reflexes.

Treatment is conducted with him sitting on a large hammock. The therapist stands in front of him and supports him bilaterally at the shoulders, maintaining protraction and external rotation. Vestibular stimulation is provided by rocking him back and forth in the swing in a slow, rhythmical manner. He laughs and smiles and increases the controlled extensor tone of his trunk. As this occurs the therapist is able to let her hands move from supporting the shoulders to support at the elbows, maintaining the protraction and external rotation at the shoulders and extension of the elbows. She continues to move the swing back and forth, and he maintains the trunk extension. The vestibular stimulation is then changed to make the situation more challenging. As the swing is gently moved from side to side, tonic extensor tone associated with a Moro reflex emerges, and he begins to lose postural control. The therapist adapts her handling, initially by stopping the side-to-side movement and providing firm proprioceptive stimulation through the elbows to inhibit the tonic extensor tone. If this is not effective, she then moves her handling back to the shoulders to provide more proximal control. As she resumes handling from this point he once again relaxes and develops controlled extension of the trunk. Thus the progression to follow is to introduce the side-to-side movement while maintaining the handling at the shoulders. When he is able to hold his controlled extensor tone in response to this vestibular input, the therapist then adapts her handling and moves to the elbows. Following a similar progression, her aim is to move to the hands, and finally to withdraw her control altogether thus achieving sensory integration.

REFERENCES

Abuladze, K. S. (1968) 'Central inhibition of reflexes and the problem of the coupled activity of cerebral hemispheres.' *Progress in Brain Research,* **22,** 3–7.
Ayres, A. J. (1972) *Sensory Integration and Learning Disorders.* Los Angeles: Western Psychological Services. pp. 1, 11, 114, 114–115.
—— (1979) *Sensory Integration and the Child.* Los Angeles: Western Psychological Services. pp. 94, 181–185.
Korner, A. F., Grobstein, R. (1966) 'Visual altertness as related to soothing in neonates: implications for maternal stimulation and deprivation.' *Child Development,* **37,** 867–876.
Prechtl, H. F. R., Beintema, D. J. (1968) Die *Neurologische Untersuchung des Reifen Neugeborenen.* Stuttgart: Georg Thieme.
Rushworth, G. (1971) 'On postural and righting reflexes.' *In:* Copp, C. B. (Ed.) *Readings in Early Development for Occupational and Physical Therapy Students.* Springfiled, Ill.: C. C. Thomas.

FURTHER READING

NEUROLOGY

Brown, D. R. (1980) *Neurosciences for Allied Health Professionals.* St Louis: C. V. Mosby.
Noback, C., Demarest, R. (1975) *The Human Nervous System—Basic Principles of Neurobiology.* New York: McGraw Hill.
Reuck, A. V. S., Knight, J. (Eds.) (1967) *Ciba Foundation Symposium: Myotatic, Kinesthetic and Vestibular Mechanisms.* London: Churchill; Boston: Little Brown.

DEVELOPMENT

Banus, B. S. (1979) *The Developmental Therapist, 2nd Edn.* Thorofare, N.J.: Charles B. Slack.
Bobath, B. (1971) 'Motor development, its effect on general development, and application to the treatment of cerebral palsy.' *Physiotherapy,* **57,** 526–532.
—— Bobath, K. (1964) 'The facilitation of normal postural reactions and movements in the treatment of cerebral palsy.' *Physiotherapy,* **50,** 246–262.
Bobath, K. (1971) 'The normal postural reflex mechanism and its deviation on children with cerebral palsy.' *Physiotherapy,* **57,** 515–525.
Brazelton, T. B. (1972) *Infants and Mothers.* New York: Dell; London: Hutchinson.
—— (1974) *Toddlers and Parents.* New York: Dell.
Ginsburg, H., Opper, S. (1969) *Piaget's Theory of Intellectual Development—an Introduction.* New Jersey: Prentice Hall.
Leboyer, F. (1976) *Loving Hands: The Traditional Indian Art of Baby Massage.* New York: Alfred Knopf.

Ayres, A. J. (1976) *The Effect of Integrative Therapy on Learning Disabled Children: Final Report of a Research Project.* Center for the Study of Sensory Integrative Dysfunction, 201 Sth Lake, Pasadena, Ca. 91101.

—— (1977) 'Effect of sensory integrative therapy on the co-ordination of children with choreoathetoid movements.' *American Journal of Occupational Therapy*, **31**, 291–293.

—— Tickle, L. S. (1980) 'Hyper-responsivity to touch and vestibular stimuli predict positive response to sensory integration procedures by autistic children'. *American Journal of Occupational Therapy*, **34**, 375–381.

Bright, T., Bittick, K., Fleeman, B. (1981) 'Reduction of self-injurious behavior using sensory integrative techniques.' *American Journal of Occupational Therapy*, **35**, 167–172.

Clark, F. A., Miller, L., Thomas, J., Kucherawy, D., Azen, S. (1978) 'A comparison of operant and sensory integrative methods on developmental parameters in profoundly retarded adults.' *American Journal of Occupational Therapy*, **32**, 86–92.

Keating, N. R. (1979) 'A comparison of duration of nystagmus as measured by the Southern California postrotary nystagmus test and electronystagmography.' *American Journal of Occupational Therapy*, **33**, 92–97.

Montgomery, P., Gauger, J. (1978) 'Sensory dysfunction in children who toe walk.' *Physical Therapy*, **58**, 1195–1204.

—— Richter, E. (1977) *Sensorimotor Integration for Developmentally Disabled Children: a Handbook.* Los Angeles: Western Psychological Services.

Ornitz, E. (1974) 'The modulation of sensory input and motor output in autistic children.' *Journal of Autism and Childhood Schizophrenia*, **4**, 197–216.

—— Forsythe, A. B., de la Pena, A. (1973) 'The effect of vestibular and auditory stimulation in the rapid eye movement of REM sleep in normal and autistic children.' *Archives of General Psychiatry*, **29**, 786–791.

—— Brown, M., Mason, A., Putnam, N. (1978) 'Effects of visual input on vestibular nystagmus in autistic children.' *Archives of General Psychiatry*, **31**, 369–375.

Pribram, K. H., McGuiness, D. (1975) 'Arousal, activation, and efforts in the control of attention.' *Psychological Review*, **32**, 116–149.

de Quiros, J. B., Schrager, O. L. (1978) *Neuropsychological Fundamentals in Learning Disabilities.* San Raphael, Ca.: Academic Therapy Publications.

8
THERAPEUTIC POSSIBILITIES IN CEREBRAL PALSY: A NEUROLOGIST'S VIEW

Lindsay McLellan

Neurologists have traditionally concentrated upon the diagnosis of disease more than on its treatment. To some extent this has reflected a pessimistic attitude to the chances of inducing recovery by medical means. Recently this stance has started to alter, partly because certain treatments have been evolved as in Parkinsonism which do require medical expertise to get right, but also because of a more widespread realisation that the management of disability is an important and intellectually rewarding activity which makes a difference to patients' ability to realise their potential and reduces the incidence of complications of their disease.

Hypotheses and proofs

The history of medicine shows that the correct theoretical explanation of a treatment has rarely pre-dated its discovery. Nevertheless, hypotheses regarding the mechanisms of a treatment are comforting to all concerned with it. Patients with pernicious anaemia 50 years ago who were treated by removal of all their teeth no doubt felt that their money had been well spent, and their dentist would have had few qualms that it had been well earned. These days we are more circumspect and empiricism is respectable, provided that the treatment really *has* been established empirically as effective. Once the clinician has proved this, basic scientists tend to become interested and sooner or later the explanation will follow.

Maturation and modelling

What is known about the development of mechanisms of movement in the normal growing child, and the ways in which various external influences can alter it? The answer is remarkably little. Physiological studies of the mechanisms involved in the brain and spinal cord have established basic wiring diagrams showing how different structures in the brain are interconnected, but the dynamics of the working system are only beginning to be understood. Even so, some principles have already been established that could be relevant to cerebral palsy.

The process of maturation of the brain of higher animals is tightly programmed in time. Though the development of neurones and many of their connections is likely to be genetically determined, the programming of each element appears to be designed to integrate with concurrent developments among its contacts. If an element is missing during the crucial period of time, that particular set of synaptic connections does not develop and, most important, cannot later be induced to do so even if the abnormal circumstances are removed. Thus the connections laid down in the occipital cortex of the kitten's brain to detect movement in the horizontal plane depend upon appropriate visual stimulation for their formation. Once the critical period of a few weeks has passed, that phase in development cannot be induced and kittens deprived of the appropriate visual input at that time can never develop it.

Another important principle is that of 'programmed cell death'. Just as a normal pattern of connections may need the appropriate pattern of activity at the right time in order to develop normally, so other systems rely upon the anticipated fall-out of some of their connections which has the effect of guiding the synaptic structure into its mature pattern. Thus each step in the process of maturation appears to depend upon the successful completion of the preceding step, but there is only a short window of time in which each step can occur and this depends upon the biological age of the neurones concerned; there is no going back.

Processes like this could explain the great difficulty of identifying cerebral palsy in infants, since the abnormalities could become apparent in a cumulative way as maturation proceeds even though the first link in the chain has perhaps been broken before the birth. How then does one explain the fact that some infants have suffered very severe damage to one cerebral hemisphere and yet grow up with little observable deficit? Clearly such damage has not altered the pattern of connections in a counterproductive way but instead provoked the development of connections that later enabled one hemisphere to control both sides of the body. The mechanisms that determine this propensity to connect for good or ill are very poorly understood but it seems unlikely that the biological clock could be put back by external influences later in life, since the neurones have by then passed the age at which they can behave in that particular way.

This is not of course to deny that new connections are made and old ones lost throughout life in response to activity in the brain. In general it seems likely that synapses that are frequently activated become consolidated and may proliferate, while failure to activate a synapse may lead to its degeneration. However, this is by no means the only way that synaptic connectivity is moulded. The response of a synapse appears to differ according to its nature, the influences upon it and the neurotransmitters involved. Trophic factors other than neurotransmitters are also implicated in long-term proliferation or degeneration of synapses.

Other shorter-term changes occur in synapses. For example, a synapse whose input is reduced or abolished may develop 'denervation hypersensitivity' due to an increase in the number of receptor sites on the post-synaptic membrane. This allows the post-synaptic membrane to respond to smaller amounts of neurotransmitter than would previously have been necessary to fire it, thus counteracting to some extent the effects of the reduced input. Other neuronal systems show responses that alter rapidly during the passage of a train of impulses.

The activity of individual synapses cannot be inferred from what one can observe in an intact animal, or in a child with cerebral palsy. The fact that spasticity gradually builds up during the early months or years of life cannot be ascribed to a particular series of events, for it could be due to a number of different mechanisms and we do not as yet have methods to identify them. For example, it could be that the sequence of pre-programmed maturation changes has been disrupted so that a series of inappropriate connections are made, or connections that were required are not made. Inactive synapses would gradually degenerate while active ones could be maintained or proliferate. It is not even known whether spasticity results from the 'unmasking' of excitatory neurones because of degeneration of inhibitory ones, or from the formation of new excitatory synaptic connections. Another factor that is important in grasping the scale of physiological theory is the fact that reflexes such as stretch responses or tactile responses may show short-term fluctuations of habituation or sensitisation which progressively diminish or increase the response to a given stimulus the longer it is repeated.

Theory and practice
For practical purposes, not enough is known about the process of maturation, or the effects of damage, or about the brain mechanisms responsible for movement to enable any predictions to be made about the effectiveness of different treatments in the management of cerebral palsy. The advantage of one treatment over another can be proved only by careful clinical evaluation. Knowledge of the neurophysiological mechanisms that could be involved is irrelevant to this process.

It could be argued that this is too sweeping a statement since the fact that the therapist believes in a mechanism may in itself be part of the treatment. The various authors contributing to this book have emphasised the complexity of the management process in enlisting the enthusiasm and motivation of the child, family and therapeutic team. Knowledge confers status, which can certainly help to maintain momentum during treatment but there is a danger that such hypotheses come to be regarded as proof of efficacy for measures that have been inadequately tested. Ultimately that can only bring the measures themselves into disrepute. Such disrepute may be entirely undeserved, such as the scepticism with which acupuncture was regarded until recently by Western medicine; for many years the unconvincing theories of acupuncture blinded us to the fact that it worked.

Cultural influences on schools of treatment
Cultural influences are worth emphasising because they could go some way to explaining the discrepancies between the different viewpoints in this book. The discrepancies are interesting and could reflect personal or cultural factors rather than error. This is alluded to by David Scrutton when he discusses the polarisation between eclectic and systems approaches. I suspect that many British therapists, or parents for that matter, would blanche at a checklist of 580 skills, intuitively pushing it to one side and rolling up their sleeves. By contrast, their opposite numbers in New York might be greatly encouraged by such an inventory. Another factor is that the British Health Service puts pressure on therapists to use their scanty resources of time as economically as possible; programmes that are funded according to the work done or the time spent are likely to be less economical with time. Such considerations do not impugn the integrity of different therapists or the effectiveness of their treatment but they do make for diversity. Diversity is to be welcomed in our present state of ignorance and is indeed to be expected when one

considers the mixture of physical, social and psychological factors that determines a successful outcome.

Common ground in therapy
More interesting and more informative than disagreement is the common ground shared by all the successful schools of treatment or management of cerebral palsy. There is general agreement that early treatment is important and that one of the things that makes this very difficult to achieve is the difficulty of diagnosing milder cases in infants, and a virtual impossibility of predicting an eventual outcome which could then serve as a goal. Improved diagnosis would certainly help management. This could come about from recent technical advances such as Nuclear Magnetic Resonance and Positron Emission Tomography scanning which for the first time allow non-invasive measurement of metabolic activity in different parts of the brain but it will be many years before today's research techniques can be validated by clinical follow-up.

The plea for early treatment is a two-edged weapon in any disorder of uncertain prognosis, since the therapy will inevitably claim credit for children who were actually normal or almost normal to start with. On the other hand, biological age seems to be important in the timing of sequences of maturation and there may be periods of time especially in the first weeks or months of life when invisible processes of maturation could be affected by specific interventions that would thereafter be ineffective. The emotional harm suffered by parents who have been incorrectly alerted to a high risk of cerebral palsy is a strong argument for careful prospective trials of any form of therapy applied to groups of children whose chances of developing cerebral palsy are small. Such treatment should not be given routinely until it has been proved effective.

Another area of shared ground is the emphasis given to motivating the child and involving the parents, in order that unwanted activities are avoided or stopped and that as much time as possible is spent in ways considered to be beneficial. Here again the extraordinary diversity of the problems encountered in cerebral palsy demands a highly individual approach; Conductive Education stands apart from the others here in its emphasis on group activities, as well as its search to avoid physically holding or supporting the child.

There is general agreement about the importance of the needs of the rest of the family including the patient's siblings. Someone has to solve the conundrum of wanting the child to think of himself and be regarded by others as a 'normal human being' while his childhood is taking up so much of the family's resources.

There do seem to me to be many areas of agreement in the various physical manoeuvres that are recommended by different schools, even though the emphasis is different. Common patterns of activity occur which can be inhibited or facilitated by various and possibly complementary means such as positioning, encouragement, passive handling, skin stimulation and verbal and visual instruction. Perhaps it is the British taste for compromise (so often mistaken for hypocrisy) that makes this encouraging rather than disturbing.

Clinical trials

Progress in these controversial areas will come most quickly through comparative trials of different aspects of the treatment and this process could be helped by the improved methods of clinical and neurophysiological assessment that are now available. No two cerebral-palsied children are identical, but one particular component of a child's disability such as flexion of the elbow could be tested without interrupting treatment for other aspects of the disorders that are present; although I appreciate that a few purists might consider that even this interferes with their treatment.

Clinical description can be augmented by physiological tests and in particular by recording of the electromyograms (EMG) from specific muscles. This information is valuable because it indicates the relative activity in protagonist and antagonist muscles, which differs considerably in passive and various active movements of a limb. The spasticity of cerebral palsy gives particularly surprising results when analysed in this way. Many patients show idiosyncratic and stereotyped patterns of activity that could not have been predicted even by careful observation. This type of analysis is used by some orthopaedic surgeons to identify patients who would benefit from tendon transfers about the foot, and also to identify which tendons should be transferred. Furthermore, EMGs have given valuable insights into the mechanism of antispastic drug treatment. Suppression of passive stretch responses can be achieved without altering in any way the patterns seen in a voluntary movement. Some patients have been found to respond not by a diminution of antagonist activity but by an increase in protagonist activity during voluntary movement.

These techniques refine clinical assessment and provide information that could be useful both diagnostically and for the purpose of follow-up. They have, of course, considerable potential for the education of therapists early in training since the trainee's skill in assessing the patient could be reinforced by studying recordings from the various muscles of the limb.

Other physiological tests are also available, many of which measure reflex responses of some kind, usually triggered by electrical stimulation applied to the skin overlying a peripheral nerve. These tests have to be interpreted very cautiously since no correlation with clinical features, response to treatment, or outcome has been established but it is possible that they will in time help to identify sub-groups of patients who respond particularly well to particular forms of treatment. Only time will tell whether they can also be used to help predict outcome.

Rôle of the therapist in research

The use of such tools will require the therapist to be part of a research team encompassing the necessary skills. The therapist must play a central rôle in such a team and it is a matter of considerable concern that by no means all therapists are familiar with research methodology or have had any training in it. In recent years new medical treatments have been tried in an attempt to improve function in established neurological disease. Chronic electrical stimulation can now be applied to the brain and spinal cord and can also be used to activate muscles directly by electrodes placed on the skin or in the muscle itself. Such measures do not yet have an accepted rôle in the management of cerebral palsy. Even when they are effective, active support from the therapy team is necessary in order to establish worthwhile gains in function.

Future developments
Physical therapies are going to continue to be the mainstay of management of cerebral palsy for the foreseeable future. Two complementary aspects— therapeutic technique, and successful negotiation of a goal that can be reached at the right cost—are vital. What advances might be made in the techniques of improving motor function in cerebral palsy? My own view is that it is unlikely that major new advances in technique will now be made intuitively by therapists in the course of their routine work. This phase in the evolution of treatment, which has contributed so much to the care of cerebral palsy in the past 40 years, has been achieved by a few outstandingly creative therapists who have developed great sensitivity and skill in assessing and monitoring the effects of their work. One of the difficulties of passing on these skills to others is the lack of detailed objective proof of efficacy. It is easier to prove a reduction in the incidence of complications, such as contractures or dislocations, than it is to prove that a patient has acquired a new skill because one cannot predict with certainty what skills would have developed without treatment. The fact that one school insists on constant handling to mould a child's movements as they develop, while another seeks to avoid any physical contact, implies that one or both methods are mistaken. Alternatively both could contain equal amounts of good and bad, in which case a mixture of both could be better than either in their pure form.

Conclusion
It is not possible to support one type of physical therapy against another on grounds of principle, since the evidence does not exist that would justify such a conclusion. Cerebral palsy is a fascinating and rewarding field in which to work and to do research, and there is plenty to be done. Each member of the management team will have his own particular skills and interests and should be able to contribute to the development of new methods and the instruction of others in their use. In the end the team must have a sense of proportion and considerable flexibility in order to succeed with every case it treats. The problems of cerebral palsy do not consist simply of a set of physical or physiological abnormalities, but a complex of social and psychological needs affecting the whole of the family which may from time to time—and for some patients all the time—require more skill and attention than the physical handicap itself.